Practice the

MW00981562

Health Occupations Aptitude Exam Practice Test Questions

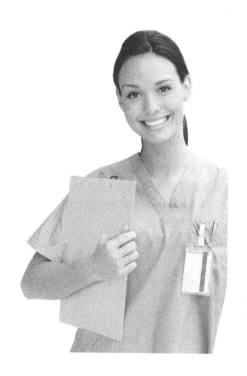

Published by

Complete **TEST**
Preparation Inc.

Copyright Notice

We strongly recommend that students check with exam providers for up-to-date information regarding test content.

ISBN-13: 978-1-928077-73-2

Version 7.0 January 2017

Published by
Complete Test Preparation Inc.
Victoria BC Canada

Visit us on the web at http://www.test-preparation.ca
Printed in the USA

About Complete Test Preparation Inc.

The Complete Test Preparation Inc. Team has been publishing high quality study materials since 2005. Thousands of students visit our websites every year, and thousands of students, teachers and parents all over the world have purchased our teaching materials, curriculum, study guides and practice tests.

Complete Test Preparation Inc. is committed to providing students with the best study materials and practice tests available on the market. Members of our team combine years of teaching experience, with experienced writers and editors, all with advanced degrees.

Feedback

We welcome your feedback. Email us at feedback@test-preparation.ca with your comments and suggestions. We carefully review all suggestions and often incorporate reader suggestions into upcoming versions. As a Print on
Demand Publisher, we update our products frequently.

Sustainability and Eco-Responsibility

Here at Complete Test Preparation, trees are valuable to the Earth and the health and wellbeing of everyone. Minimizing our ecological footprint and effect on the environment, we choose CreateSpace, an eco-responsible printing company.

Electronic routing of our books reduces greenhouse gas emissions, worldwide. When a book order is received, the order is filled at the printing location closest to the client. Using environmentally friendly publishing technology, of the Espresso book printing machine, Complete Test Preparation are printed as they are requested, saving thousands of books, and trees over time. This process offers the stable and viable alternative keeping healthy sustainability of our environment.

 Find us on Facebook

www.facebook.com/CompleteTestPreparation

Contents

Getting Started

CONGRATULATIONS! By deciding to take the Health Occupations Aptitude Examination (PSB or HOAE) , you have taken the first step toward a great future! Of course, there is no point in taking this important examination unless you intend to do your best to earn the highest grade you possibly can. That means getting yourself organized and discovering the best approaches, methods and strategies to master the material. Yes, that will require real effort and dedication on your part, but if you are willing to focus your energy and devote the study time necessary, before you know it you will be opening that letter of acceptance to the nursing school of your dreams.

We know that taking on a new endeavour can be a little scary, and it is easy to feel unsure of where to begin. That's where we come in. These practice tests are designed to help you improve your test-taking skills, show you a few tricks of the trade and increase both your competency and confidence.

Note, however, that the makers of the PSB may have changed the types of questions on the exam as well as exam content after this study guide was created. We recommend that you check with the creators of the test for any new information, and be sure to read the materials supplied on registration carefully.

What is on the PSB

The PSB has these sections: vocabulary, arithmetic, spelling, reading comprehension, form relations and natural sciences. Since how well you score in each of these areas will determine whether or not you get into the best nursing school possible, it is important to be prepared.

Part I - Academic Aptitude

Verbal Sub-test

The Verbal Sub-test contains 30 vocabulary related questions.

Arithmetic Sub-test

The Arithmetic Sub-test contains 30 questions on basic arithmetic.

Nonverbal Sub-test

The Nonverbal Sub-test contains 30 questions that test your comprehension of form relations and ability to manipulate shapes mentally.

Part II – Spelling

This section contains around 30 spelling questions.

Part III - Reading Comprehension

This section contains questions based on a short passage. The questions test comprehension, making inferences and conclusions.

Part IV – Natural Sciences

The section covers introductory level biology, chemistry, and natural science.

The PSB Study Plan

Now that you have made the decision to take the PSB, it is time to get started. Before you do another thing, you will need to figure out a plan of attack. The very best study tip is to start early! The longer the time period you devote to regular study practice, the more likely you will be to retain the material and be able to access it quickly. If you thought that 1x20 is the same as 2x10, guess what? It really is not, when it comes to study time. Reviewing material for just an hour per day over the course of 20 days is far better than studying for two hours a day for only 10 days. The more often you revisit a particular piece of information, the better you will know it. Not only will your grasp and understanding be better, but your ability to reach into your brain and quickly and efficiently pull out the tidbit you need, will be greatly enhanced as well.

The great Chinese scholar and philosopher Confucius believed that true knowledge could be defined as knowing both what you know and what you do not know. The first step in preparing for the PSB® Exam is to assess your strengths and weaknesses. You may already have an idea of what you know and what you do not know, but evaluating yourself using our Self-Assessment modules for each of the three areas, math, english science and reading, will clarify the details.

Making a Study Schedule

To make your study time most productive you will need to develop a study plan. The purpose of the plan is to organize all the bits of pieces of information in such a way that you will not feel overwhelmed. Rome was not built in a day, and learning everything you will need to know to pass the PSB® Exam is going to take time, too. Arranging the material you need to learn into manageable chunks is the best way to go. Each study session should make you feel as though you have succeeded in accomplishing your goal, and your goal is simply to learn what you planned to learn during that particular session. Try to organize the content in such a way that each study session builds upon previous ones. That way, you will retain the information, be better able to access it, and review the previous bits and pieces at the same time.

Exam Component	Rate from 1 - 5
Vocabulary	
Arithmetic	
Spelling	
Nonverbal	

Reading Comprehension	
Passage Comprehension	
Drawing inferences & conclusions	
Natural Sciences	
Biology	
Chemistry	
General Science	

Making a Study Schedule

The key to making a study plan is to divide the material you need to learn into manageable size and learn it, while at the same time reviewing the material that you already know.

Using the table above, any scores of three or below, you need to spend time learning, going over, and practicing this subject area. A score of four means you need to review the material, but you don't have to spend time re-learning. A score of five and you are OK with just an occasional review before the exam.

A score of zero or one means you really do need to work on this and you should allocate the most time and give it the highest priority. Some students prefer a 5-day plan and others a 10-day plan. It also depends on how much time you have until the exam.

Here is an example of a 5-day plan based on an example from the table above:

Vocabulary: 1   Study 1 hour everyday – review on last day

Arithmetic: 3   Study 1 hour for 2 days then ½ hour a day, then review

Spelling: 4   Review every second day

Biology: 2 Study 1 hour on the first day – then ½ hour everyday

Reading Comprehension: 5   Review for ½ hour every other day

Basic Science: 5   Review for ½ hour every other day

It makes sense to focus your study time on those subjects where you need the most work but unless you create a visual chart for yourself, chances are good you will get confused in no time. First, write out what you need to study and how much time you want to devote to it. Next, consider how many days you have before the test. Plan to take time off from studying on the day before the exam is scheduled. On the last day before the test, you will not learn anything and will probably only confuse yourself. Besides, giving yourself a little break means you will feel fresher on the day of the test.

Make a table that includes slots for the number of days before the test and the number of hours you have available to study each day. We suggest working with half-hour and one-hour time slots; less than that means you will get set up to study and it will be time to quit, and more than an hour might result in mental fatigue.

Now you are ready to begin filling in the blanks. Give the most time to those subjects you need to study the most. It is also a good idea to assign your weakest subjects the most regular time slots. In fact, even just thirty minutes a day will help lock in the information you need. Of course, those subjects that you know like the back of your hand can be assigned the shortest blocks of time. You will note in the chart we have created that a half hour two or three times a week is all you will need for your strongest subjects.

If you have between two and three hours a day in which to study, you might create a chart that looks something like this to help yourself stay organized:

Day	Subject	Time
Monday		
Study	Vocabulary	1 hour
Study	Biology	1 hour
	½ hour break	
Study	Arithmetic	1 hour
Review	Spelling	½ hour
Tuesday		
Study	Vocabulary	1 hour
Study	Biology	½ hour
	½ hour break	
Study	Arithmetic	½ hour
Review	Spelling	½ hour
Review	Basic Science	½ hour
Wednesday		
Study	Vocabulary	1 hour
Study	Biology	½ hour
	½ hour break	
Study	Arithmetic	½ hour
Review	Basic Science	½ hour
Thursday		
Study	Vocabulary	½ hour
Study	Biology	½ hour
Review	Arithmetic	½ hour
	½ hour break	
Review	Basic Science	½ hour
Review	Spelling	½ hour
Friday		
Review	Vocabulary	½ hour
Review	Biology	½ hour
Review	Arithmetic	½ hour
	½ hour break	
Review	Spelling	½ hour
Review	Biology	½ hour

Tips for making a schedule

Once you set a schedule that works, stick with it! Establish study sessions that are realistic. Blocking out study time that is too long or too short means you will be tempted to cheat. Instead, schedule study sessions that are reasonable and you will set yourself up for success!

Schedule breaks. Breaks are just as important as study time. Work out a rotation of studying and brief breaks that works for you.

Build up study time. If you find it hard to sit still and study for an hour at first, build up to it. Start with 20 minutes, and then take a break. Once you get used to 20-minute study sessions, increase the time to 30 minutes. Gradually work your way up to a full hour.

40 minutes to an hour is optimal. Studying for longer is unlikely to be productive. Studying for periods that are too short won't give you enough time to really learn anything.

Approach math differently. Studying math is different than studying other subjects because you use a different part of your brain. The best way to study math is to practice every day. This will train your mind to think in a mathematical way. If you miss a day or two, the mathematical mind-set is gone and you have to start all over again to build it up.

Practice Test 1

Part 1 - Academic Aptitude

Verbal Sub-test – Vocabulary
Questions: 30
Time: 30 Minutes

Mathematics Sub-test
Questions: 30
Time: 30 Minutes

Nonverbal Sub-test
Questions: 30
Time: 30 Minutes

Part II – Spelling
Questions: 30
Time: 30 Minutes

Part III – Reading Comprehension
Questions: 35
Time: 35 Minutes

Part VI – Basic Science
Questions: 60
Time: 60 minutes

The practice test portion presents questions that are representative of the type of question you should expect to find on the PSB. However, they are not intended to match exactly what is on the PSB. Don't worry though! If you can answer these questions, you will have not trouble with the PSB.

For the best results, take this Practice Test as if it were the real exam. Set aside time when you will not be disturbed, and a location that is quiet and free of distractions. Read the instructions carefully, read each question carefully, and answer to the best of your ability.

Use the bubble answer sheets provided. When you have completed the Practice Test, check your answer against the Answer Key and read the explanation provided.

Part 1 – Vocabulary Sub-test

	A	B	C	D	E			A	B	C	D	E
1	○	○	○	○	○		21	○	○	○	○	○
2	○	○	○	○	○		22	○	○	○	○	○
3	○	○	○	○	○		23	○	○	○	○	○
4	○	○	○	○	○		24	○	○	○	○	○
5	○	○	○	○	○		25	○	○	○	○	○
6	○	○	○	○	○		26	○	○	○	○	○
7	○	○	○	○	○		27	○	○	○	○	○
8	○	○	○	○	○		28	○	○	○	○	○
9	○	○	○	○	○		29	○	○	○	○	○
10	○	○	○	○	○		30	○	○	○	○	○
11	○	○	○	○	○							
12	○	○	○	○	○							
13	○	○	○	○	○							
14	○	○	○	○	○							
15	○	○	○	○	○							
16	○	○	○	○	○							
17	○	○	○	○	○							
18	○	○	○	○	○							
19	○	○	○	○	○							
20	○	○	○	○	○							

Part I – Mathematics Sub-test

	A	B	C	D	E			A	B	C	D	E
1	○	○	○	○	○		21	○	○	○	○	○
2	○	○	○	○	○		22	○	○	○	○	○
3	○	○	○	○	○		23	○	○	○	○	○
4	○	○	○	○	○		24	○	○	○	○	○
5	○	○	○	○	○		25	○	○	○	○	○
6	○	○	○	○	○		26	○	○	○	○	○
7	○	○	○	○	○		27	○	○	○	○	○
8	○	○	○	○	○		28	○	○	○	○	○
9	○	○	○	○	○		29	○	○	○	○	○
10	○	○	○	○	○		30	○	○	○	○	○
11	○	○	○	○	○							
12	○	○	○	○	○							
13	○	○	○	○	○							
14	○	○	○	○	○							
15	○	○	○	○	○							
16	○	○	○	○	○							
17	○	○	○	○	○							
18	○	○	○	○	○							
19	○	○	○	○	○							
20	○	○	○	○	○							

Part I – Nonverbal Sub-test

	A	B	C	D	E			A	B	C	D	E
1	○	○	○	○	○		21	○	○	○	○	○
2	○	○	○	○	○		22	○	○	○	○	○
3	○	○	○	○	○		23	○	○	○	○	○
4	○	○	○	○	○		24	○	○	○	○	○
5	○	○	○	○	○		25	○	○	○	○	○
6	○	○	○	○	○		26	○	○	○	○	○
7	○	○	○	○	○		27	○	○	○	○	○
8	○	○	○	○	○		28	○	○	○	○	○
9	○	○	○	○	○		29	○	○	○	○	○
10	○	○	○	○	○		30	○	○	○	○	○
11	○	○	○	○	○
12	○	○	○	○	○
13	○	○	○	○	○
14	○	○	○	○	○
15	○	○	○	○	○
16	○	○	○	○	○
17	○	○	○	○	○
18	○	○	○	○	○
19	○	○	○	○	○
20	○	○	○	○	○

Answer Sheet - Part II – Spelling

	A	B	C	D	E		A	B	C	D	E
1	○	○	○	○	○	21	○	○	○	○	○
2	○	○	○	○	○	22	○	○	○	○	○
3	○	○	○	○	○	23	○	○	○	○	○
4	○	○	○	○	○	24	○	○	○	○	○
5	○	○	○	○	○	25	○	○	○	○	○
6	○	○	○	○	○	26	○	○	○	○	○
7	○	○	○	○	○	27	○	○	○	○	○
8	○	○	○	○	○	28	○	○	○	○	○
9	○	○	○	○	○	29	○	○	○	○	○
10	○	○	○	○	○	30	○	○	○	○	○
11	○	○	○	○	○						
12	○	○	○	○	○						
13	○	○	○	○	○						
14	○	○	○	○	○						
15	○	○	○	○	○						
16	○	○	○	○	○						
17	○	○	○	○	○						
18	○	○	○	○	○						
19	○	○	○	○	○						
20	○	○	○	○	○						

Part III – Reading Comprehension

	A	B	C	D	E		A	B	C	D	E
1	○	○	○	○	○	21	○	○	○	○	○
2	○	○	○	○	○	22	○	○	○	○	○
3	○	○	○	○	○	23	○	○	○	○	○
4	○	○	○	○	○	24	○	○	○	○	○
5	○	○	○	○	○	25	○	○	○	○	○
6	○	○	○	○	○	26	○	○	○	○	○
7	○	○	○	○	○	27	○	○	○	○	○
8	○	○	○	○	○	28	○	○	○	○	○
9	○	○	○	○	○	29	○	○	○	○	○
10	○	○	○	○	○	30	○	○	○	○	○
11	○	○	○	○	○	31	○	○	○	○	○
12	○	○	○	○	○	32	○	○	○	○	○
13	○	○	○	○	○	33	○	○	○	○	○
14	○	○	○	○	○	34	○	○	○	○	○
15	○	○	○	○	○	35	○	○	○	○	○
16	○	○	○	○	○						
17	○	○	○	○	○						
18	○	○	○	○	○						
19	○	○	○	○	○						
20	○	○	○	○	○						

Part IV - Natural Sciences

	A B C D E		A B C D E
1	○ ○ ○ ○ ○	31	○ ○ ○ ○ ○
2	○ ○ ○ ○ ○	32	○ ○ ○ ○ ○
3	○ ○ ○ ○ ○	33	○ ○ ○ ○ ○
4	○ ○ ○ ○ ○	34	○ ○ ○ ○ ○
5	○ ○ ○ ○ ○	35	○ ○ ○ ○ ○
6	○ ○ ○ ○ ○	36	○ ○ ○ ○ ○
7	○ ○ ○ ○ ○	37	○ ○ ○ ○ ○
8	○ ○ ○ ○ ○	38	○ ○ ○ ○ ○
9	○ ○ ○ ○ ○	39	○ ○ ○ ○ ○
10	○ ○ ○ ○ ○	40	○ ○ ○ ○ ○
11	○ ○ ○ ○ ○	41	○ ○ ○ ○ ○
12	○ ○ ○ ○ ○	42	○ ○ ○ ○ ○
13	○ ○ ○ ○ ○	43	○ ○ ○ ○ ○
14	○ ○ ○ ○ ○	44	○ ○ ○ ○ ○
15	○ ○ ○ ○ ○	45	○ ○ ○ ○ ○
16	○ ○ ○ ○ ○	46	○ ○ ○ ○ ○
17	○ ○ ○ ○ ○	47	○ ○ ○ ○ ○
18	○ ○ ○ ○ ○	48	○ ○ ○ ○ ○
19	○ ○ ○ ○ ○	49	○ ○ ○ ○ ○
20	○ ○ ○ ○ ○	50	○ ○ ○ ○ ○
21	○ ○ ○ ○ ○	51	○ ○ ○ ○ ○
22	○ ○ ○ ○ ○	52	○ ○ ○ ○ ○
23	○ ○ ○ ○ ○	53	○ ○ ○ ○ ○
24	○ ○ ○ ○ ○	54	○ ○ ○ ○ ○
25	○ ○ ○ ○ ○	55	○ ○ ○ ○ ○
26	○ ○ ○ ○ ○	56	○ ○ ○ ○ ○
27	○ ○ ○ ○ ○	57	○ ○ ○ ○ ○
28	○ ○ ○ ○ ○	58	○ ○ ○ ○ ○
29	○ ○ ○ ○ ○	59	○ ○ ○ ○ ○
30	○ ○ ○ ○ ○	60	○ ○ ○ ○ ○

Part 1 – Academic Aptitude

Vocabulary Sub-test

Directions: For each question below, select the word that is most different in meaning.

1. a. Torture b. Martyr c. Excruciate d. Torment

2. a. Quip b. Joke c. Jest d. Jaunty

3. a. Lodge b. Accommodate c. Billet d. Reside

4. a. Radiate b. Stellate c. Emanate d. Conciliate

5. a. Coquette b. Philander c. Romance d. Rebuff

6. a. Quixotic b. Romantic c. Amorous d. Loving

7. a. Lugubrious b. Languid c. Slow d. Laborious

LOL

wth

8. a. Renegotiate b. Reconcile c. Harmonize d. Conciliate

9. a. Sanction b. Authorize c. Proscribe d. Approve

10. a. Progenitor b. Ancestor c. Antecedent d. Descendant

11. a. Conformist b. Iconoclast c. Maverick d. Unorthodox

12. a. Indolence b. Laziness c. Lugubrious d. Cheerful

13. a. Vulgar b. Decent c. Tasteless d. Brash

14. a. Unrelenting b. Ceaseless c. Constant d. Intermittent

15. a. Derision b. Scornful c. Approval d. Approbation

16. a. Roguishly b. Truthfully c. Dishonorably d. Disloyally

17. a. Giddiness b. Light-headedness c. Vertigo d. Phobia

18. a. Persistent b. Docile c. Pertinacious d. Tenacious

19. a. Boisterous b. Placid c. Rambunctious d. Rumbustious

20. a. Specious b. Spurious c. Legitimate d. Inauthentic

21. a. Invidious b. Discriminatory c. Unfavorable d. Apprehensible

22. a. Osculate b. Share c. Kiss d. Defalcate

23. a. Lie b. Veracity c. Mendacity d. Truth

24. a. Facet b. Feature c. Angle d. Whole

25. a. Negligent b. Discerning c. Prescient d. Discriminating

26. a. Venerate b. Esteem c. Disdain d. Prize

27. a. Redeemable b. Corrigible c. Amendable d. Catharsis

28. a. Raucous b. Noisy c. Orderly d. Obstreperous

29. a. Averse b. Loath c. Antipathetic d. Agreeable

30. a. Rampant b. Controlled c. Uncontrolled d. Abundant

Mathematics Sub-test

1. What is 1/3 of 3/4?

    a. 1/4
    b. 1/3
    c. 2/3
    d. 3/4

2. Susan wants to buy a leather jacket that costs $545.00 and is on sale for 10% off. What is the approximate cost?

    a. $525

    b. $450

    c. $475

    d. $500

3. 3.14 + 2.73 + 23.7 =

    a. 28.57 ←

    b. 30.57

    c. 29.56

    d. 29.57

4. Express 0.27 + 0.33 as a fraction.

    a. a. 3/6

    b. 4/7

    c. 3/5

    d. 2/7

5. A woman spent 15% of her income on an item and ends up with $120. What percentage of her income is left?

    a. 12%

    b. 85%

    c. 75% ←

    d. 95%

6. 8 is what percent of 40?

    a. 10%

    b. 15%

    c. 20%

    d. 25%

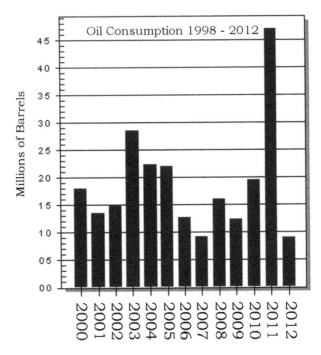

7. The graph above shows oil consumption in millions of barrels for the period, 1998 - 2012. What year did oil consumption peak?

    a. 2011

    b. 2010

    c. 2008

    d. 2009

8. Translate the following into an equation: 2 + a number divided by 7.

    a. (2 + X)/7

    b. (7 + X)/2

    c. (2 + 7)/X

    d. 2/(7 + X)

9. .4% of 36 is

    a. 1.44

    b. .144

    c. 14.4

    d. 144

10. The physician ordered 5 mg Coumadin; 10 mg/tablet is on hand. How many tablets will you give?

    a. .5 tablet

    b. 1 tablet

    c. .75 tablet

    d. 1.5 tablets

11. The physician ordered 20 mg Tylenol/kg of body weight; on hand is 80 mg/tablet. The child weighs 12 kg. How many tablets will you give?

    a. 1 tablet

    b. 3 tablets

    c. 2 tablets

    d. 4 tablets

12. What number is MCMXC?

a. 1990

b. 1980

c. 2000

d. 1995

13. Consider the following population growth chart.

Country	Population 2000	Population 2005
Japan	122,251,000	128,057,000
China	1,145,195,000	1,341,335,000
United States	253,339,000	310,384,000
Indonesia	184,346,000	239,871,000

What country is growing the fastest?

a. Japan

b. China

c. United States

d. Indonesia

14. If y = 4 and x = 3, solve yx^3

a. -108

b. 108

c. 27

d. 4

15. Convert 16 quarts to gallons.

    a. 1 gallons

    b. 8 gallons ✓

    c. 4 gallons

    d. 4.5 gallons

16. Convert 45 kg. to pounds.

    a. 10 pounds

    b. 100 pounds

    c. 1,000 pounds

    d. 110 pounds

17. Translate the following into an equation: three plus a number times 7 equals 42.

    a. $7(3 + X) = 42$

    b. $3(X + 7) = 42$

    c. $3X + 7 = 42$

    d. $(3 + 7)X = 42$

18. In a class of 83 students, 72 are present. What percent of the students are absent? Provide answer up to two significant digits.

    a. 12%

    b. 13%

    c. 14%

    d. 15%

19. 5x+2(x+7) = 14x – 7. Find x

    a. 1

    b. 2

    c. 3

    d. 4

20. 5(z+1) = 3(z+2) + 11. Z=?

    a. 2

    b. 4

    c. 6

    d. 12

21. The price of a book went up from \$20 to \$25. What percent did the price increase?

    a. 5%

    b. 10%

    c. 20%

    d. 25%

22. A boy is given 2 apples while his sister is given 8 oranges. What is the ratio between the boy's apples and her oranges?

    a. 1:2

    b. 2:4

    c. 1:4

    d. 2:1

23. In the time required to serve 43 customers, a server breaks 2 glasses and slips 5 times. The next day, the same server breaks 10 glasses. How many customers did she serve?

    a. 25

    b. 43

    c. 86

    d. 215

24. A square lawn has an area of 62,500 square meters. What is the cost of building fence around it at a rate of $5.5 per meter?

    a. $4000

    b. $4500

    c. $5000

    d. $5500

25. Solve for n, when 5n + (19 – 2) = 67.

    a. 21

    b. 10

    c. 15

    d. 7

26. Below is the attendance for a class of 45.

Day	Number of Absent Students
Monday	5
Tuesday	9
Wednesday	4
Thursday	10
Friday	6

What is the average attendance for the week?

    a. 88%

    b. 85%

    c. 81%

    d. 77%

27. A distributor purchased 550 kilograms of potatoes for $165. He distributed these at a rate of $6.4 per 20 kilograms to 15 shops, $3.4 per 10 kilograms to 12 shops and the remainder at $1.8 per 5 kilograms. If his total distribution cost is $10, what will his profit be?

    a. $8.60

    b. $24.60

    c. $14.90

    d. $23.40

28. How much pay does Mr. Johnson receive if he gives half of his pay to his family, $250 to his landlord, and has exactly 3/7 of his pay left over?

    a. $3600

    b. $3500

    c. $2800

    d. $1750

29. A boy has 4 red, 5 green and 2 yellow balls. He chooses two balls randomly. What is the probability that one is red and other is green?

    a. 2/11

    b. 19/22

    c. 20/121

    d. 9/11

30. The cost of waterproofing canvas is .50 a square yard. What's the total cost for waterproofing a canvas truck cover that is 15' x 24'?

    a. $18.00

    b. $6.67

    c. $180.00

    d. $20.00

Nonverbal Sub-test

1.

2.

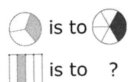

is to

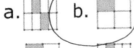

is to ?

a. 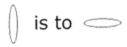 b.

c. d.

3.

is to

is to ?

a. b.

c. d.

4.

is to

is to ?

a. b.

c. d.

5.

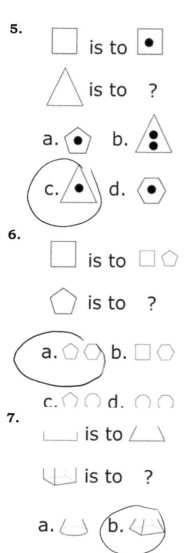

□ is to ⊡

△ is to ?

a. ⬠● b. △(two dots)

c. (◯ around △●) d. ⬡●

6.

□ is to □ ⬠

⬠ is to ?

a. (⬠ ⬡ circled) b. □ ⬡

c. ⬠ ◯ d. ◯ ◯

7.

⌐ is to ◿

⊔ is to ?

a. ◠ b. (◿ circled)

c. ⊔ d. ◿

8.

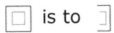 is to ⌐

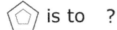 is to   ?

a. ⟩   b. ⟩⟩

c. ⟩   d. ⌐

9.   ☐ is to ⌐

⬠ is to   ?

a.)   b. ⟩

c.)   d. ⌐

10. Consider the following sequence:

+ * + * | * + * + | * * + * | + + __ __

a. + *
b. * *
c. + +
d. * +

**Directions: Choose the option that completes a relation-
ship that is the same as the relationship in the first pair.**

11. Acting : Theater :: Gambling :

    a. Gym

    b. Bar

    c. Club

    d. Casino

12. Pork : Pig :: Beef :

    a. Herd

    b. Farmer

    c. Cow

    d. Lamb

13. Fruit : Banana :: Mammal :

    a. Cow

    b. Snake

    c. Fish

    d. Sparrow

14. Slumber : Sleep :: Bog :

    a. Dream

    b. Foray

    c. Swamp

    d. Night

15. Zoology : Animals

    a. Ecology : Pollution
    b. Botany : Plants   *Study of*
    c. Chemistry : Atoms
    d. History : People

16. Child : Human

    a. Dog : Pet
    b. Kitten : Cat
    c. Cow : Milk
    d. Bird : Robin

17. Wax : Candle

    a. Ink : Pen
    b. Clay : Bowl   *← made of itself*
    c. String : Kite
    d. Liquid : Cup

18. Which word does not belong with the others?

    a. Jet
    b. Float plane
    c. Kite
    d. Biplane

19. Which of the following does not belong?

    a. Number
    b. Denominate   *} Synonyms*
    c. Numerate
    d. Figure

20. Which of the following does not belong?

a. Abc

b. bCD

c. Nmo

d. Pqr

21. Which of the following does not belong?

a. CD

b. OP

c. LM

d. BD

22. Which of the following does not belong?

a. 121212

b. 141414

c. 151415

d. 292929

23. Which of the following does not belong?

a. 246

b. 123

c. 468

d. 024

24. Which of the following does not belong?

a. QRS

b. LMN

c. ACF

d. RST

25. Which of the following does not belong?

    a. aBCd

    b. lMNo

    c. PQRs

    d. tUVw

26. Which of the following does not belong?

    a. ABCD

    b. JKLM

    c. PQRS   no vow als

    d. WXYZ

27. Which of the following does not belong?

    a. BBCCDDEE

    b. LLMMNNOO

    c. HHIIJJKK

    d. RRSSTTUU

28. Which of the following does not belong?

    a. 123

    b. 246

    c. 456

    d. 789

29. Which of the following does not belong?

    a. def

    b. nop   vowel

    c. tuv

    d. lmn

30. Which of the following does not belong?

a. Argue

b. Talk

c. Dispute

d. Contest

Part II – Spelling

1. Choose the correct spelling.

a. Realy

b. Reelly

c. Really

d. None of the Above

2. Choose the correct spelling.

a. Rescede

b. Receede

c. Reacede

d. Recede

3. Choose the correct spelling.

a. Refrense

b. Refrence

c. Reference

d. Refference

4. Choose the correct spelling.

    a. Similar
    b. Similiar
    c. Simillar
    d. Semilar

5. Choose the correct spelling.

    a. Sking
    b. Skying
    c. Skiing
    d. Skinng

6. Choose the correct spelling.

    a. Stregth
    b. Stregth
    c. Strength
    d. Strenth

7. Choose the correct spelling.

    a. Technical
    b. Tecknical
    c. Techical
    d. Teknical

8. Choose the correct spelling.

    a. Theries
    b. Theories
    c. Theorys
    d. Theorries

9. Choose the correct spelling.

a. Possess

b. Posese

c. Posess

d. Poses

10. Choose the correct spelling.

a. Portrey

b. Portray

c. Potray

d. Porttray

11. Choose the correct spelling.

a. Proceadure

b. Proceedure

c. Procedure

d. Procedrure

12. Choose the correct spelling.

a. Proceed

b. Proced

c. Procead

d. Procceed

13. Choose the correct spelling.

a. Profresor

b. Proffessor

c. Profesor

d. Professor

14. Choose the correct spelling.

  a. Persue

  b. Pursu

  c. Pursue

  d. Porsue

15. Choose the correct spelling.

  a. Realice

  b. Realize

  c. Relise

  d. None of the Above

16. Choose the correct spelling.

  a. Peice

  b. Pece

  c. Piece

  d. Peece

17. Choose the correct spelling.

  a. Posibel

  b. Posible

  c. Possible

  d. None of the Above

18. Choose the correct spelling.

  a. Encouraging

  b. Encuraging

  c. Encuoraging

  d. None of the Above

19. Choose the correct spelling.

    a. Harras

    b. Harasse

    c. Harass

    d. Haress

20. Choose the correct spelling.

    a. Manetain

    b. Maintain

    c. Maintane

    d. Manetane

21. Choose the correct spelling.

    a. Hieght

    b. Height

    c. Heit

    d. Heigt

22. Choose the correct spelling.

    a. Heross

    b. Heros

    c. Herose

    d. Heroes

23. Choose the correct spelling.

    a. Geneus

    b. Genius

    c. Ginius

    d. Gennius

24. Choose the correct spelling.

    a. Incedentally

    b. Incidentaly

    c. Incidentally

    d. Incidentilly

25. Choose the correct spelling.

    a. Parallel

    b. Parallell

    c. Paralel

    d. Parralel

26. Choose the correct spelling.

    a. Absenes

    b. Absence

    c. Absense

    d. Absennce

27. Choose the correct spelling.

    a. Advurtisement

    b. Advertisment

    c. Advertisement

    d. Advertesement

28. Choose the correct spelling.

    a. Bileif

    b. Bilief

    c. Beleif

    d. Belief

29. Choose the correct spelling.

a. Comparative
b. Comperative
c. Comparetive
d. Conparative

30. Choose the correct spelling.

a. Definately
b. Definitely
c. Definetely
d. Difenitely

Reading Comprehension.

Questions 1 – 4 refer to the following passage.

Passage 1 - Infectious Disease

An infectious disease is a clinically evident illness resulting from the presence of pathogenic agents, such as viruses, bacteria, fungi, protozoa, multi-cellular parasites, and unusual proteins known as prions. Infectious pathologies are also called communicable diseases or transmissible diseases, due to their potential of transmission from one person or species to another by a replicating agent (as opposed to a toxin).

Transmission of an infectious disease can occur in many different ways. Physical contact, liquids, food, body fluids, contaminated objects, and airborne inhalation can all transmit infecting agents.

Transmissible diseases that occur through contact with an ill person, or objects touched by them, are especially infective, and are sometimes called contagious diseases. Communicable diseases that require a more specialized route of infection, such as through blood or needle transmission, or sexual transmission, are usually not regarded as contagious.

The term infectivity describes the ability of an organism to enter, survive and multiply in the host, while the infectious-ness of a disease indicates the comparative ease with which the disease is transmitted. An infection however, is not syn-onymous with an infectious disease, as an infection may not cause important clinical symptoms. [1]

1. What can we infer from the first paragraph in this passage?

  a. Sickness from a toxin can be easily transmitted from one person to another.

  b. Sickness from an infectious disease can be easily transmitted from one person to another.

  c. Few sicknesses are transmitted from one person to another.

  d. Infectious diseases are easily treated.

2. What are two other names for infections' pathologies?

  a. Communicable diseases or transmissible diseases

  b. Communicable diseases or terminal diseases

  c. Transmissible diseases or preventable diseases

  d. Communicative diseases or unstable diseases

3. What does infectivity describe?

  a. The inability of an organism to multiply in the host

  b. The inability of an organism to reproduce

  c. The ability of an organism to enter, survive and mul-tiply in the host

  d. The ability of an organism to reproduce in the host

4. How do we know an infection is not synonymous with an infectious disease?

a. Because an infectious disease destroys infections with enough time.

b. Because an infection may not cause important clinical symptoms or impair host function.

c. We do not. The two are synonymous.

d. Because an infection is too fatal to be an infectious disease.

Questions 5 – 8 refer to the following passage.

Passage 2 - Virus

A virus (from the Latin virus meaning toxin or poison) is a small infectious agent that can replicate only inside the living cells of other organisms. Most viruses are too small to be seen directly with a microscope. Viruses infect all types of organisms, from animals and plants to bacteria and single-celled organisms.

Unlike prions and viroids, viruses consist of two or three parts: all viruses have genes made from either DNA or RNA, all have a protein coat that protects these genes, and some have an envelope of fat that surrounds them when they are outside a cell. (Viroids do not have a protein coat and prions contain no RNA or DNA.) Viruses vary from simple to very complex structures. Most viruses are about one hundred times smaller than an average bacterium. The origins of viruses in the evolutionary history of life are unclear: some may have evolved from plasmids—pieces of DNA that can move between cells—while others may have evolved from bacteria.

Viruses spread in many ways; plant viruses are often transmitted from plant to plant by insects that feed on sap, such as aphids, while animal viruses can be carried by blood-sucking insects. These disease-bearing organisms are known as vectors. Influenza viruses are spread by coughing and sneezing. HIV is one of several viruses transmitted through sexual contact and by exposure to infected blood. Viruses can infect only a limited range of host cells called the "host range." This can be broad as, when a virus is capable of infecting many species or narrow. [2]

5. What can we infer from the first paragraph in this selection?

    a. A virus is the same as bacterium

    b. A person with excellent vision can see a virus with the naked eye

    c. A virus cannot be seen with the naked eye

    d. Not all viruses are dangerous

6. What types of organisms do viruses infect?

    a. Only plants and humans

    b. Only animals and humans

    c. Only disease-prone humans

    d. All types of organisms

7. How many parts do prions and viroids consist of?

    a. Two

    b. Three

    c. Either less than two or more than three

    d. Less than two

8. What is one common virus spread by coughing and sneezing?

    a. AIDS

    b. Influenza

    c. Herpes

    d. Tuberculosis

Questions 9 – 11 refer to the following passage.

Passage 3 – Thunderstorms

The first stage of a thunderstorm is the cumulus stage, or developing stage. In this stage, masses of moisture are lifted upwards into the atmosphere. The trigger for this lift can be insulation heating the ground producing thermals, areas where two winds converge, forcing air upwards, or where winds blow over terrain of increasing elevation. Moisture in the air rapidly cools into liquid drops of water, which appears as cumulus clouds.

As the water vapor condenses into liquid, latent heat is released which warms the air, causing it to become less dense than the surrounding dry air. The warm air rises in an updraft through the process of convection (hence the term convective precipitation). This creates a low-pressure zone beneath the forming thunderstorm. In a typical thunderstorm, about 5×10^8 kg of water vapor is lifted, and the quantity of energy released when this condenses is about equal to the energy used by a city of 100,000 in a month. [3]

9. The cumulus stage of a thunderstorm is the

    a. The last stage of the storm

    b. The middle stage of the storm formation

    c. The beginning of the thunderstorm

    d. The period after the thunderstorm has ended

10. One of the ways the air is warmed is

    a. Air moving downwards, which creates a high-pressure zone

    b. Air cooling and becoming less dense, causing it to rise

    c. Moisture moving downward toward the earth

    d. Heat created by water vapor condensing into liquid

11. Identify the correct sequence of events

a. Warm air rises, water droplets condense, creating more heat, and the air rises farther.

b. Warm air rises and cools, water droplets condense, causing low pressure.

c. Warm air rises and collects water vapor, the water vapor condenses as the air rises, which creates heat, and causes the air to rise farther.

d. None of the above.

Questions 12 – 14 refer to the following passage.

Passage 4 – US Weather Service

The United States National Weather Service classifies thunderstorms as severe when they reach a predetermined level. Usually, this means the storm is strong enough to inflict wind or hail damage. In most of the United States, a storm is considered severe if winds reach over 50 knots (58 mph or 93 km/h), hail is ¾ inch (2 cm) diameter or larger, or if meteorologists report funnel clouds or tornadoes. In the Central Region of the United States National Weather Service, the hail threshold for a severe thunderstorm is 1 inch (2.5 cm) in diameter. Though a funnel cloud or tornado indicates the presence of a severe thunderstorm, the various meteorological agencies would issue a tornado warning rather than a severe thunderstorm warning.

Meteorologists in Canada define a severe thunderstorm as either having tornadoes, wind gusts of 90 km/h or greater, hail 2 centimeters in diameter or greater, rainfall more than 50 millimeters in 1 hour, or 75 millimeters in 3 hours.

Severe thunderstorms can develop from any type of thunderstorm. [4]

12. What is the purpose of this passage?

a. Explaining when a thunderstorm turns into a tornado

b. Explaining who issues storm warnings, and when these warnings should be issued

c. Explaining when meteorologists consider a thunderstorm severe

d. None of the above

13. It is possible to infer from this passage that

a. Different areas and countries have different criteria for determining a severe storm

b. Thunderstorms can include lightning and tornadoes, as well as violent winds and large hail

c. If someone spots both a thunderstorm and a tornado, meteorological agencies will immediately issue a severe storm warning

d. Canada has a much different alert system for severe storms, with criteria that are far less

14. What would the Central Region of the United States National Weather Service do if hail was 2.7 cm in diameter?

a. Not issue a severe thunderstorm warning.

b. Issue a tornado warning.

c. Issue a severe thunderstorm warning.

d. Sleet must also accompany the hail before the Weather Service will issue a storm warning.

Question 15 refers to the following Table of Contents.

Contents

15. Consider the table of contents above. What page would you find information about natural selection and adaptation?

　　a. 81

　　b. 90

　　c. 110

　　d. 132

Questions 16 – 19 refer to the following passage.

Passage 5 – Clouds

A cloud is a visible mass of droplets or frozen crystals float-ing in the atmosphere above the surface of the Earth or other planetary bodies. Another type of cloud is a mass of material in space, attracted by gravity, called interstellar clouds and nebulae. The branch of meteorology which studies clouds is called nephrology. When we are speaking of Earth clouds, wa-ter vapor is usually the condensing substance, which forms small droplets or ice crystal. These crystals are typically 0.01 mm in diameter. Dense, deep clouds reflect most light, so they appear white, at least from the top. Cloud droplets scatter light very efficiently, so the farther into a cloud light travels, the weaker it gets. This accounts for the gray or dark appearance at the base of large clouds. Thin clouds may appear to have acquired the color of their environment or background. [4]

16. What are clouds made of?

    a. Water droplets.

    b. Ice crystals.

    c. Ice crystals and water droplets.

    d. Clouds on Earth are made of ice crystals and water droplets.

17. The main idea of this passage is

    a. Condensation occurs in clouds, having an intense effect on the weather on the surface of the earth.

    b. Atmospheric gases are responsible for the gray color of clouds just before a severe storm happens.

    c. A cloud is a visible mass of droplets or frozen crystals floating in the atmosphere above the surface of the Earth or other planetary body.

    d. Clouds reflect light in varying amounts and degrees, depending on the size and concentration of the water droplets.

18. The branch of meteorology that studies clouds is called

    a. Convection

    b. Thermal meteorology

    c. Nephology

    d. Nephelometry

19. Why are clouds white on top and grey on the bottom?

a. Because water droplets inside the cloud do not reflect light, it appears white, and the farther into the cloud the light travels, the less light is reflected making the bottom appear dark.

b. Because water droplets outside the cloud reflect light, it appears dark, and the farther into the cloud the light travels, the more light is reflected making the bottom appear white.

c. Because water droplets inside the cloud reflects light, making it appear white, and the farther into the cloud the light travels, the more light is reflected making the bottom appear dark.

d. None of the above.

Questions 20 - 23 refer to the following recipe.

Who Was Anne Frank?

You may have heard mention of the word Holocaust in your History or English classes. The Holocaust took place from 1939-1945. It was an attempt by the Nazi party to purify the human race, by eliminating Jews, Gypsies, Catholics, homosexuals and others they deemed inferior to their "perfect" Aryan race. The Nazis used Concentration Camps, which were sometimes used as Death Camps, to exterminate the people they held in the camps. One of the saddest facts about the Holocaust was the over one million children under the age of sixteen died in a Nazi concentration camp. Just a few weeks before World War II was over, Anne Frank was one of those children to die.

Before the Nazi party began its persecution of the Jews, Anne Frank had a happy live. She was born in June of 1929. In June of 1942, for her 13th birthday, she was given a simple present which would go onto impact the lives of millions of people around the world. That gift was a small red diary that she called Kitty. This diary was to become

Anne's most treasured possession when she and her family hid from the Nazi's in a secret annex above her father's office building in Amsterdam.

For 25 months, Anne, her sister Margot, her parents, another family, and an elderly Jewish dentist hid from the Nazis in this tiny annex. They were never permitted to go outside, and their food and supplies were brought to them by Miep Gies and her husband, who did not believe in the Nazi persecution of the Jews. It was a very difficult life for young Anne and she used Kitty as an outlet to describe her life in hiding. After 2 years, Anne and her family were betrayed and arrested by the Nazis. To this day, nobody is exactly sure who betrayed the Frank family and the other annex residents. Anne, her mother, and her sister were separated from Otto Frank, Anne's father. Then, Anne and Margot were separated from their mother. In March of 1945, Margot Frank died of starvation in a Concentration Camp. A few days later, at the age of 15, Anne Frank died of typhus. Of all the people who hid in the Annex, only Otto Frank survived the Holocaust.

Otto Frank returned to the Annex after World War II. It was there that he found Kitty, filled with Anne's thoughts and feelings about being a persecuted Jewish girl. Otto Frank had Anne's diary published in 1947 and it has remained continuously in print ever since. Today, the diary has been published in over 55 languages and more than 24 million copies have been sold around the world. The Diary of Anne Frank tells the story of a brave young woman who tried to see the good in all people.

20. From the context clues in the passage, the word Annex most nearly means?

    a. Attic

    b. Bedroom

    c. Basement

    d. Kitchen

21. Why do you think Anne's diary has been published in 55 languages?

    a. So everyone could understand it.

    b. So people around the world could learn more about the horrors of the Holocaust.

    c. Because Anne was Jewish but hid in Amsterdam and died in Germany.

    d. Because Otto Frank spoke many languages.

22. From the description of Anne and Margot's deaths in the passage, what can we assume typhus is?

    a. The same as starving to death.

    b. An infection the Germans gave to Anne.

    c. A disease Anne caught in the concentration camp.

    d. Poison gas used by the Germans to kill Anne.

23. In the third paragraph, what does the word outlet most nearly mean?

    a. A place to plug things into the wall

    b. A store where Miep bought cheap supplies for the Frank family

    c. A hiding space similar to an Annex

    d. A place where Anne could express her private thoughts.

Questions 24 – 25 refer to the following email.

SUBJECT: MEDICAL STAFF CHANGES

To all staff:

This email is to advise you of a paper on recommended medical staff changes has been posted to the Human Resources website.

The contents are of primary interest to medical staff, other staff may be interested in reading it, particularly those in medical support roles.

The paper deals with several major issues:

1. Improving our ability to attract top quality staff to the hospital, and retain our existing staff. These changes will make our position and departmental names internationally recognizable and comparable with North American and North Asian departments and positions.

2. Improving our ability to attract top quality staff by introducing greater flexibility in the departmental structure.

3. General comments on issues to be further discussed in relation to research staff.

The changes outlined in this paper are significant. I encourage you to read the document and send to me any comments you may have, so that it can be enhanced and improved.

Gordon Simms
Administrator,
Seven Oaks Regional Hospital

24. Are all hospital staff required to read the document posted to the Human Resources website?

a. Yes all staff are required to read the document.

b. No, reading the document is optional.

c. Only medical staff are required to read the document.

d. none of the above are correct.

25. Have the changes to medical staff been made?

   a. Yes, the changes have been made.

   b. No, the changes are only being discussed.

   c. Some of the changes have been made.

   d. None of the choices are correct.

Questions 26 – 29 refer to the following passage.

Passage 6 – Navy Seals

The United States Navy's Sea, Air and Land Teams, commonly known as Navy SEALs, are the U.S. Navy's principle special operations force, and a part of the Naval Special Warfare Command (NSWC) as well as the maritime component of the United States Special Operations Command (USSOCOM).

The unit's acronym ("SEAL") comes from their capacity to operate at sea, in the air, and on land – but it is their ability to work underwater that separates SEALs from most other military units in the world. Navy SEALs are trained and have been deployed in a wide variety of missions, including direct action and special reconnaissance operations, unconventional warfare, foreign internal defence, hostage rescue, counter-terrorism and other missions. All SEALs are members of either the United States Navy or the United States Coast Guard.

In the early morning of May 2, 2011 local time, a team of 40 CIA-led Navy SEALs completed an operation to kill Osama bin Laden in Abbottabad, Pakistan about 35 miles (56 km) from Islamabad, the country's capital. The Navy SEALs were part of the Naval Special Warfare Development Group, previously called "Team 6." President Barack Obama later confirmed the death of bin Laden. The unprecedented media coverage raised the public profile of the SEAL community, particularly the counter-terrorism specialists commonly known as SEAL Team 6. [5]

26. Are Navy SEALs part of USSOCOM?

a. Yes

b. No

c. Only for special operations

d. No, they are part of the US Navy

27. What separates Navy SEALs from other military units?

a. Belonging to NSWC

b. Direct action and special reconnaissance operations

c. Working underwater

d. Working for other military units in the world

28. What other military organizations do SEALs belong to?

a. The US Navy

b. The Coast Guard

c. The US Army

d. The Navy and the Coast Guard

29. What other organization participated in the Bin Laden raid?

a. The CIA

b. The US Military

c. Counter-terrorism specialists

d. None of the above

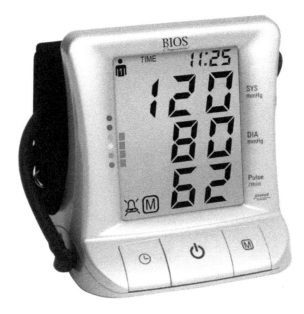

30. Consider the blood pressure gauge above. According to this gauge, what is the patient's pulse?

    a. 120 beats per minute

    b. 80 beats per minute

    c. 62 beats per minute

    d. The pulse is not shown

Questions 31 – 33 refer to the following passage.

Passage 7 - Was Dr. Seuss A Real Doctor?

A favorite author for over 100 years, Theodor Seuss Geisel was born on March 2, 1902. Today, we celebrate the birthday of the famous "Dr. Seuss" by hosting Read Across America events throughout the month of March. School children around the country celebrate the "Doctor's" birthday by making hats, giving presentations and holding read aloud circles featuring some of Dr. Seuss' most famous books.

But who was Dr. Seuss? Did he go to medical school? Where was his office? You may be surprised to know that Theodor Seuss Geisel was not a medical doctor at all. He took on the nickname Dr. Seuss when he became a noted children's book author. He earned the nickname because people said his books were "as good as medicine." All these years later, his nickname has lasted and he is known as Dr. Seuss all across the world.

Think back to when you were a young child. Did you ever want to try "green eggs and ham.?" Did you try to "Hop on Pop?" Do you remember learning about the environment from a creature called The Lorax? Of course, you must recall one of Seuss' most famous characters; that green Grinch who stole Christmas. These stories were all written by Dr. Seuss and featured his signature rhyming words and letters. They also featured made up words to enhance his rhyme scheme and even though many of his characters were made up, they sure seem real to us today.

And what of his "signature" book, The Cat in the Hat? You must remember that cat and Thing One and Thing Two from your childhood. Did you know that in the early 1950's there was a growing concern in America that children were not becoming avid readers? This was, book publishers thought, because children found books dull and uninteresting. An intelligent publisher sent Dr. Seuss a book of words that he thought all children should learn as young readers. Dr. Seuss wrote his famous story The Cat in the Hat, using those words. We can see, over the decades, just how much influence his writing has had on very young children. That is why we celebrate this doctor's birthday each March.

31. What does the word "avid" mean in the last paragraph?

    a. Good

    b. Interested

    c. Slow

    d. Fast

32. What can we infer from the statement " His books were like medicine?"

     a. His books made people feel better

     b. His books were in doctor's office waiting rooms

     c. His books took away fevers

     d. His books left a funny taste in readers' mouths.

33. Why is the publisher in the last paragraph referred to as "intelligent?"

     a. The publisher knew how to read.

     b. The publisher knew kids did not like to read.

     c. The publisher knew Dr. Seuss would be able to create a book that sold well.

     d. The publisher knew that Dr. Seuss would be able to write a book that would get young children interested in reading.

Save the Children

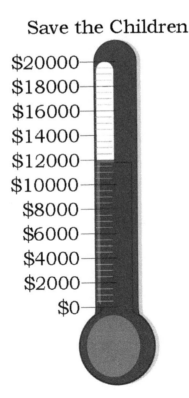

34. Consider the graphic above. The Save the Children fund has a fund-raising goal of $20,000. Approximately how much of their goal have they achieved?

    a. 3/5

    b. 3/4

    c. 1/2

    d. 1/3

35. Consider the graphic above. The Save the Children fund has a fund-raising goal of $16,000. Approximately how much of their goal have they achieved?

    a. 3/5

    b. 3/4

    c. 1/2

    d. 1/3

Section IV – Basic Science

1. Describe the differences between genotypes and phenotypes

    a. Phenotype refers to observed properties of an organism and genotype refers to the genes of an organism.

    b. Genotype refers to observed properties of an organism and phenotype refers to the genes of an organism.

    c. Phenotype refers to the DNA of an organism and genotype refers to the genes of an organism.

    d. Genotype refers to the DNA of an organism and phenotype refers to the genes of an organism.

2. A solution with a pH value of greater than 7 is

    a. Base

    b. Acid

    c. Neutral

    d. None of the above

3. Eukaryotic and prokaryotic cells are

a. Both organelles

b. Eukaryotic are not organelles

c. Both have DNA

d. Both have single membrane compartments

4. When we say that important traits for scientific classification are homologous, "homologous" means

a. Being shared among two or more animals with the same parent.

b. Being coincidentally shared by two totally different creatures.

c. Being inherited by the organisms' common ancestors.

d. Mutating beyond all reasonable expectations.

5. The manner in which instructions for building proteins, the basic structural molecules of living material, are written in the DNA is

a. Genotypic assignment

b. Chromosome pattern

c. Genetic code

d. Genetic fingerprinting

6. A _____ is a unit of inherited material, encoded by a strand of DNA and transcribed by RNA.

a. Allele

b. Phenotype

c. Gene

d. Genotype

7. Which, if any, of the following statements about meiosis are correct?

a. During meiosis, the number of chromosomes in the cell are halved.

b. Meiosis only occurs in eukaryotic cells.

c. Meiosis is the part of the life cycle that involves sexual reproduction.

d. All of these statements are correct.

8. A population of wolves expanded exponentially after a hunting ban. Within a few generations, their habitat exceeded its

a. Carrying capacity

b. Food source

c. Population limit

d. Supply capability

9. When a pouch in the large intestine becomes inflamed, this becomes an affliction known as

a. Diverticulosis

b. Diverticulitis

c. Acid Reflux

d. Colon Cancer

10. Why is detection of pathogens complicated?

a. They evolve so quickly

b. They die so quickly

c. They are invisible

d. They multiply so quickly

11. Photosynthesis is:

a. The process by which plants generate oxygen from carbon dioxide.

b. The process by which plants generate carbon dioxide from oxygen.

c. The process by which plants generate carbon dioxide and oxygen.

d. None of the above.

12. Which, if any, of the following statements are false?

a. A mutation is a permanent change in the DNA sequence of a gene.

b. Mutations in a gene's DNA sequence can alter the amino acid sequence of the protein encoded by the gene.

c. Mutations in DNA sequences usually occur spontaneously.

d. Mutations in DNA sequences can be caused by exposure to environmental agents such as sunshine.

13. Starting with the weakest, arrange the fundamental forces of nature in order of strength.

a. Gravity, Weak Nuclear Force, Electromagnetic Force, Strong Nuclear Force

b. Weak Nuclear Force, Gravity, Electromagnetic Force, Strong Nuclear Force

c. Strong Nuclear Force, Weak Nuclear Force, Electromagnetic Force, Gravity

d. Gravity, Strong Nuclear Force, Weak Nuclear Force, Electromagnetic Force

14. _____, which refers to the repeatability of measurement, does not require knowledge of the correct or true value.

    a. Precision

    b. Value

    c. Certainty

    d. Accuracy

15. Artificial selection:

    a. Is a process where desirable traits are systematically bred

    b. Is a process where traits become more or less common in a population

    c. Is a process where behaviors are favored

    d. None of the above.

16. Which of the following are not examples of vaporization?

    a. Boiling

    b. Evaporation

    c. Condensation

    d. All of the above

17. Describe the periodic table.

    a. The periodic table is a tabular display of the chemical compounds organized on the basis of their atomic numbers, electron configurations, and recurring chemical properties.

    b. The periodic table is a tabular display of the chemical elements, organized on the basis of their atomic numbers, electron configurations, and recurring chemical properties.

    c. The periodic table is a tabular display of the chemical subatomic particles, organized on the basis of their atomic numbers, electron configurations, and recurring chemical properties.

    d. None of the above.

18. **In terms of the scientific method, the term _____ refers to the act of noticing or perceiving something and/or recording a fact or occurrence.**

   a. Observation

   b. Diligence

   c. Perception

   d. Control

19. **What is the difference, of any, between kinetic energy and potential energy?**

   a. Kinetic energy is the energy of a body that results from heat while potential energy is the energy possessed by an object that is chilled

   b. Kinetic energy is the energy of a body that results from motion while potential energy is the energy possessed by an object by virtue of its position or state, e.g., as in a compressed spring.

   c. There is no difference between kinetic and potential energy; all energy is the same.

   d. Potential energy is the energy of a body that results from motion while kinetic energy is the energy possessed by an object by virtue of its position or state, e.g., as in a compressed spring.

20. **What is the sequence of developmental stages through which members of a given species must pass?**

   a. Life cycle

   b. Life expectancy

   c. Life sequence

   d. None of the above

21. Which one of the following best describes the function of a cell membrane?

a. It controls the substances entering and leaving the cell.

b. It keeps the cell in shape.

c. It controls the substances entering the cell.

d. It supports the cell structures

22. Which of these is not a rank within the area of classification or taxonomy?

a. Species

b. Family

c. Genus

d. Relative position

23. The scientific term _____ refers to a practical test designed with the intention that its results be relevant to a particular theory or set of theories.

a. Procedure

b. Variable

c. Hypothesis

d. Experiment

24. Substances that deactivate catalysts are called

a. Inhibitors

b. Catalytic poisons

c. Positive catalysts

d. None of the above

25. Describe kinetic energy.

    a. Kinetic energy is the energy an object possesses due to its mass.

    b. Kinetic energy is the energy an object possesses due to its motion.

    c. Kinetic energy is the energy an object possesses due to its chemical properties.

    d. Kinetic energy is the stored energy an object possesses.

26. The interval of confidence around the measured value such that the measured value is certain not to lie outside this stated interval refers to the _____ of that value.

    a. Accuracy

    b. Error

    c. Uncertainty

    d. Measurement

27. What are the differences, if any, between arteries, veins, and capillaries?

    a. Veins carry oxygenated blood away from the heart, arteries return oxygen-depleted blood to the heart, and capillaries are thin-walled blood vessels in which gas/ nutrient/ waste exchange occurs.

    b. Capillaries carry oxygenated blood away from the heart, veins return oxygen-depleted blood to the heart, and capillaries are thin-walled blood vessels in which gas/ nutrient/ waste exchange occurs.

    c. There are no differences; all perform the same function in different parts of the body.

    d. Arteries carry oxygenated blood away from the heart, veins return oxygen-depleted blood to the heart, and capillaries are thin-walled blood vessels in which gas/ nutrient/ waste exchange occurs.

28. What part of the body initiates inhalation?

    a. The lungs

    b. The diaphragm

    c. The larynx

    d. The kidneys

29. Another term for biological classification is:

    a. Darwinian classification.

    b. Animal classification.

    c. Molecular classification.

    d. Scientific classification.

30. What type of gene is not expressed as a trait unless inherited by both parents?

    a. Principal gene

    b. Latent gene

    c. Recessive gene

    d. Dominant gene

31. What is an approximation or simulation of a real system that omits all but the most essential variables of the system.

    a. Scientific method

    b. Independent variable

    c. Control group

    d. Scientific model

32. Neutrons are necessary within an atomic nucleus because:

    a. They bind with protons via nuclear force

    b. They bind with nuclei via nuclear force

    c. They bind with protons via electromagnetic force

    d. They bind with nuclei via electromagnetic force

33. Which of the following statements are false?

    a. Most enzymes are proteins

    b. Enzymes are catalysts

    c. Most enzymes are inorganic

    d. Enzymes are large biological molecules

34. _____ are compounds that contain hydrogen, can dissolve in water to release hydrogen ions into solution, and, in an aqueous solution, can conduct electricity.

    a. Caustics

    b. Bases

    c. Acids

    d. Salts

35. What are the basic structural units of nucleic acids (DNA or RNA) whose sequence determines individual hereditary characteristics?

    a. Gene

    b. Nucleotide

    c. Phosphate

    d. Nitrogen base

36. List the classifications of organisms in order of size.

a. Genus, Kingdom, Phylum/division, Class, Order, and Family Species

b. Order, Kingdom, Phylum/division, Genus, Class, and Family Species

c. Genus, Kingdom, Phylum/division, Class, Order, and Family Species

d. Kingdom ,Genus, Phylum/division, Class, Order, and Family Species

e. Family species, Order, Class, Phylum/division, Kingdom, and Genus

37. Where does digestion begin?

a. In the throat

b. In the stomach

c. In the intestines

d. In the mouth

38. What are the main components of the circulatory system?

a. The heart, veins and blood vessels

b. The heart, brain, and ears

c. The nose, throat and ears

d. The lungs, stomach, and kidneys

39. What is an example of a pathogen that the immune system detects?

a. An atom

b. A molecule

c. A vitamin

d. A virus

40. Explain chemical bonds.

   a. Chemical bonds are attractions between atoms that form chemical substances containing two or more atoms.

   b. Chemical bonds are attractions between protons that form chemical elements containing two or more atoms.

   c. Chemical bonds are two or more atoms that form chemical substances.

   d. None of the above

41. Which of these is not an example of a function of the stomach in digestion?

   a. Storing food

   b. Cleansing food of impurities

   c. Mixing food with digestive juices

   d. Transferring food into the intestines

42. The exchange of oxygen for carbon dioxide takes place in the alveolar area of _____.

   a. The throat

   b. The ears

   c. The appendix

   d. The lungs

43. The number of protons in the nucleus of an atom is the

   a. Atomic mass

   b. Atomic weight

   c. Atomic number

   d. None of the above

44. Natural selection is:

a. A process where biological traits become more common in a population

b. A process where biological traits become less common in a population

c. A process where biological traits become more or less common in a population

d. None of the above

45. Sex chromosomes are designated as being "X" or "Y" chromosomes. In terms of sex chromosomes, what differences exist between males and females?

a. Females have two X chromosomes and males have one X chromosome and one Y chromosome.

b. Females have one X chromosome, and males have one X chromosome and one Y chromosome.

c. Females have one Y chromosome, while males have one X chromosome.

d. Females have one X chromosome and one Y chromosome, and males have two X chromosomes.

46. How does the immune system fight off disease?

a. By identifying and killing tumor cells and pathogens.

b. By creating new blood cells that fight disease.

c. By expelling infection through the blood stream.

d. By giving you energy to resist disease infections.

47. Identify the chemical properties of water.

a. Water has two hydrogen atoms covalently bonded to one oxygen atom

b. Water has two oxygen atoms covalently bonded to one hydrogen atom

c. Water has two hydrogen atoms polar covalently bonded to one oxygen atom

d. Water has two oxygen atoms polar covalently bonded to one hydrogen atom

48. Which of the following is not true of atomic theory?

a. Originated in the early 19th century with the work of John Dalton.

b. Is the field of physics that describes the characteristics and properties of atoms that make up matter.

c. Explains temperature as the momentum of atoms.

d. Explains macroscopic phenomenon through the behavior of microscopic atoms.

49. A condition in which the heart beats too fast, too slow, or with an irregular beat is called _____.

a. Hypertension

b. Angina

c. Cardiac arrest

d. Arrythmia

50. The best way to avoid most digestive diseases is _____.

a. Eating a healthy diet

b. Eating only proteins

c. Never eating dessert

d. Trying not to get angry

51. An example of an important side-benefit of the respiratory system is

a. The air allows whistling.

b. The oxygen expelled can be recycled for other uses.

c. The air being expelled from the mouth allows for speaking.

d. The air expelled from the body also expels disease and germs.

52. An example of a disease of the lungs that is caused or made worse by smoking is

    a. Emphysema

    b. Strep throat

    c. Muscular dystrophy

    d. Leukemia

53. What is an example of an early response by the immune system to infection?

    a. Inhalation

    b. Inflammation

    c. Respiration

    d. Exhalation

54. Which cells are an important weapon in the fight against infection?

    a. Red blood cells

    b. White blood cells

    c. Barrier cells

    d. Virus cells

55. The complementary bases found in DNA are _____ and _____ or _____ and _____.

    a. Adenine and thymine or cytosine and guanine

    b. Cytosine and thymine or adenine and guanine

    c. Adenine and cytosine or thymine and guanine

    d. None of the above

56. The full complement of genes carried by a single set of chromosomes is a _____.

a. Genome

b. Genetics

c. Genetic code

d. Gene amplification

57. _____ is a classification of organisms into different categories based on their physical characteristics and presumed natural relationship.

a. Biology

b. Taxonomy

c. Grouping

d. Nomenclature

57. What is the order of hierarchy of levels in the biological classification of organisms?

a. Kingdom, phylum, class, order, family, genus, and species

b. Phylum, kingdom, class, order, family, genus, and species

c. Order, phylum, class, kingdom, family, genus, and species

d. Kingdom, phylum, order, class, family, genus, and species

59. What is any compound produced by a chemical reaction between a base and an acid?

a. Salt

b. Radical

c. Crystal

d. Electrolyte

60. What is a graphical description of feeding relation-ships among species in an ecological community.

    a. Food web

    b. Food chain

    c. Food network

    d. Food sequence

Answer Key

Vocabulary

1. B

2. D

3. D

4. D

5. D

6. A

7. D

8. A

9. C

10. D

11. A

12. D

13. B

14. D

15. C

16. B

17. D

18. B

19. B

20. C

21. D

22. D

23. A

24. D

25. A

26. C

27. D

28. C

29. D

30. B

Math Answer Key

1. A
1/3 X 3/4 = 3/12 = 1/4
To multiply fractions, multiply the numerator and denominator.

2. D
The question asks for approximate cost, so work with round numbers. The jacket costs $545.00 so we can round up to $550. 10% of $550 is 55. We can round down to $50, which is easier to work with. $550 - $50 is $500. The jacket will cost about $500.

The actual cost will be 10% X 545 = $54.50
545 – 54.50 = $490.50

3. D
3.14 + 2.73 = 5.87 and 5.87 + 23.7 = 29.57

4. C
To convert a decimal to a fraction, take the places of decimal

as your denominator, here 2, so in 0.27, '7' is in the 100th place, so the fraction is 27/100 and 0.33 becomes 33/100.

Next estimate the answer quickly to eliminate obvious wrong choices. 27/100 is about 1/4 and 33/100 is 1/3. 1/3 is slightly larger than 1/4, and 1/4 + 1/4 is 1/2, so the answer will be slightly larger than 1/2.

Looking at the choices, choice A can be eliminated since 3/6 = 1/2. Choice D, 2/7 is less than 1/2 and be eliminated. The answer is going to be choice B or choice C.
Do the calculation, 0.27 + 0.33 = 0.60 and 0.60 = 60/100 = 3/5, Choice C is correct.
5. B
Spent 15% - 100% - 15% = 85%

6. C
This is an easy question, and shows how you can solve some questions without doing the calculations. The question is, 8 is what percent of 40. Take easy percentages for an approximate answer and see what you get.

10% is easy to calculate because you can drop the zero, or move the decimal point. 10% of 40 = 4, and 8 = 2 X 4, so, 8 must be 2 X 10% = 20%.

Here are the calculations which confirm the quick approximation.
8/40 = X/100 = 8 * 100 / 40X = 800/40 = X = 20

7. A
According to the graph, oil consumption peaked in 2011.

8. A
2 + a number divided by 7.
(2 + X) divided by 7.
(2 + X)/7

9. B
.4/100 * 36 = .4 * 36/100 = .144

10. A

5 mg/10/mg X 1 tab/1 = .5 tablets

11. B

Step 1: Set up the formula to calculate the dose to be given in mg as per weight of the child:-
Dose ordered X Weight in Kg = Dose to be given
Step 2: 20 mg X 12 kg = 240 mg
240 mg/80 mg X 1 tab/1 = 240/80 = 3 tablets

12. A

MCMXC is 1990. 1000 + (1000 − 100) + (100 − 10) = 1990

13. D

Indonesia is growing the fastest at about 30%.

14. B

$(4)(3^3) = (4)(27) = 108$

15. C

4 quarts = 1 gallon, 16 quarts = 16/4 = 4 gallons.
Conversion problems are easy to get confused. One way to think of them is which is larger - quarts or gallons?   Gallons are larger, so if you are converting from quarts to gallons the number of gallons will be a smaller number. Keeping that in mind, you can do a 'common-sense' check on your answer.

16. B

0.45 kg = 1 pound, 1 kg. = 1/0.45 and 45 kg = 1/0.45 x 45 = 99.208, or 100 pounds.

17. C

Three plus a number times 7 equals 42. Let X be the number.
(3 + X) times 7 = 42
7(3 + X) = 42

18. B

Number of absent students = 83 − 72 = 11

Percentage of absent students is found by proportioning the number of absent students to total number of students in the class = 11•100/83 = 13.25

Checking the answers, we round 13.25 to the nearest whole number: 13%

19. C
To solve for x, first simplify the equation
5x + 2x + 14 = 14x – 7
7x + 14 = 4x -7
7x – 14x + 14 = -7
7x – 14x = -7 – 14
-7x = -21
x = -21/-7
x=3

20. C
5z + 5 = 3z +6 + 11
5z -3z + 5 =6 + 11
5z – 3z = 6 + 11 -5
2z = 17 – 5
2z = 12
z= 12/2
z= 6

21. D
Price increased by $5 ($25-$20). to calculate the percent increase:
5/20 = X/100
500 = 20X
X = 500/20
X = 25%

22. C
The ratio is 2 to 8, or 1:4.

23. D
2 glasses are broken for 43 customers so 1 glass breaks for every 43/2 customers served, therefore 10 glasses implies 43/2 x 10=215. She served 215 customers.

24. D
As the lawn is square shaped, the length of one side will be the square root of the area. $\sqrt{62,500}$ = 250 meters. So, the perimeter is found by 4 times the length of the side of the

square:

250 * 4 = 1000 meters.

Since each meter costs $5.5, the total cost of the fence will be 1000 * 5.5 = $5,500.

25. B
5n + (19 – 2) = 67, 5n + 17 = 67, 5n = 67 -17, 5n = 50, n = 50/5 = 10

26. B

Day	Absent	Present	% Attendance
Monday	5	40	88.88%
Tuesday	9	36	80.00%
Wednesday	4	41	91.11%
Thursday	10	35	77.77%
Friday	6	39	86.66%

Sum of the percent attendance is 424.42. Divide by 5 for the average, 424.42/5 = 84.884. Round up to 85%.

27. B
The distribution is done in three different rates and amounts:

$6.4 per 20 kilograms to 15 shops … 20•15 = 300 kilograms distributed

$3.4 per 10 kilograms to 12 shops … 10•12 = 120 kilograms distributed

550 - (300 + 120) = 550 - 420 = 130 kilograms left. This amount is distributed by 5 kilogram portions. So, this means that there are 130/5 = 26 shops.

$1.8 per 130 kilograms.

We need to find the amount he earned overall these distributions.

$6.4 per 20 kilograms : 6.4•15 = $96 for 300 kilograms

$3.4 per 10 kilograms : 3.4•12 = $40.8 for 120 kilograms

$1.8 per 5 kilograms : 1.8•26 = $46.8 for 130 kilograms

So, he earned 96 + 40.8 + 46.8 = $ 183.6

The total distribution cost is given as $10

The profit is found by: Money earned - money spent ... It is important to remember that he bought 550 kilograms of potatoes for $165 at the beginning:

Profit = 183.6 - 10 - 165 = $8.6

28. B
We check the fractions taking place in the question. We see that there is a "half" (that is 1/2) and 3/7. So, we multiply the denominators of these fractions to decide how to name the total money. We say that Mr. Johnson has 14x at the beginning; he gives half of this, meaning 7x, to his family. $250 to his landlord. He has 3/7 of his money left. 3/7 of 14x is equal to:

14x•(3/7) = 6x

So,

Spent money is: 7x + 250

Unspent money is: 6x

Total money is: 14x

We write an equation: total money = spent money + unspent money

14x = 7x + 250 + 6x

14x - 7x - 6x = 250

x = 250

We are asked to find the total money that is 14x:

$14x = 14 \cdot 250 = \$3500$

29. A
The probability that the 1st ball drawn is red = 4/11
The probability that the 2nd ball drawn is green = 5/10
The combined probability will then be 4/11 X 5/10 =
20/110 = 2/11

30. D
First calculate total square feet, which is 15•24 = 360 ft2.
Next, convert this vaue to square yards, (1 yards2 = 9 ft2)
which is 360/9 = 40 yards2. At $0.50 per square yard, the
total cost is 40•0.50 = $20.

Section III – Nonverbal

1. D
The relation is the same figure rotated.

2. D
The shaded area is divided in half in the second figure.

3. D
The relation is the same figure rotated to the right.

4. B
The relation is the number of dots is one-half the number of
sides.

5. C
The pattern is the same figure with a dot inside.

6. A
The relation is the same figure smaller, plus another figure
with one more side.

7. B
The relation is the bottom half of the figure.

8. C
The relation is the right half of the first object.

9. B
The relation is the right half of the first object.

10. D
Each time the * and + alternate, either singly or doubles.

11. D
This is a place relationship. Acting is done in a theater in the same way gambling is done in a casino.

12. C
Pork is the meat of a pig in the same way beef is the meat of a cow.

13. A
This is a classification relationship. The first is the class which the second belongs.

14. C
Slumber is a synonym for sleep and bog is a synonym for swamp.

15. B
The first is the study of the second. Zoology is the study of animals in the same way botany is the study of plants.

16. B
This is a type relationship. A child is a young human just as a kitten is a young cat.

17. B
This is a composition relationship. A candle is made of wax and a bowl is made of clay.

18. C
A kite is not a type of plane.

19. D
This is a relationship of words question. All the choices are synonyms of count, except figure.

20. B
This is a capital small letter relationship. All choices start with a capital letter.

21. D
BD is not a sequence of consecutive letters.

22. C
This is a repetition pattern. All the choices repeat a 2-letter sequence.

23. B
123 are consecutive, the others are obtained by adding 2.

24. C
ACF is not a sequence of consecutive letters.

25. C
Capital small letter relationship. All choices have the middle two letters capitalized except c.

26. A
This is a vowel and consonant relationship. All the choices are only consonants, except Choice A.

27. C
This is a vowel and consonant relationship. All the choices have 2 vowels at the end.

28. B
246 is not a sequence of consecutive numbers.

29. D
This is a vowel and consonant relationship. All the choices have one vowel in the middle position.

30. B
This is a word meaning relationship. Talk is not a synonym for any of the choices.

Part II – Spelling

1. C
2. D
3. C
4. A
5. C
6. C
7. A
8. B
9. A
10. B
11. C
12. A
13. D
14. C
15. B
16. C
17. C
18. A
19. C
20. B
21. B
22. D
23. B
24. C
25. A
26. B
27. C
28. D
29. A
30. B

Section III – Reading Comprehension

1. B

We can infer from this passage that sickness from an infectious disease can be easily transmitted from one person to another.

From the passage, "Infectious pathologies are also called communicable diseases or transmissible diseases, due to their potential of transmission from one person or species to another by a replicating agent (as opposed to a toxin)."

2. A

Two other names for infectious pathologies are communicable diseases and transmissible diseases.

From the passage, "Infectious pathologies are also called communicable diseases or transmissible diseases, due to their potential of transmission from one person or species to another by a replicating agent (as opposed to a toxin)."

3. C

Infectivity describes the ability of an organism to enter, survive and multiply in the host. This is taken directly from the passage, and is a definition type question.

Definition type questions can be answered quickly and easily by scanning the passage for the word you are asked to define.

"Infectivity" is an unusual word, so it is quick and easy to scan the passage looking for this word.

4. B

We know an infection is not synonymous with an infectious disease because an infection may not cause important clinical symptoms or impair host function.

5. C

We can infer from the passage that, a virus is too small to be seen with the naked eye. Clearly, if they are too small to be seen with a microscope, then they are too small to be seen with the naked eye.

6. D

Viruses infect all types of organisms. This is taken directly from the passage, "Viruses infect all types of organisms, from animals and plants to bacteria and single-celled organisms."

7. C

The passage does not say exactly how many parts prions and viroids consist of. It does say, "Unlike prions and viroids, viruses consist of two or three parts ..." so we can infer they consist of either less than two or more than three parts.

8. B
A common virus spread by coughing and sneezing is Influenza.

9. C
The cumulus stage of a thunderstorm is the beginning of the thunderstorm.

This is taken directly from the passage, "The first stage of a thunderstorm is the cumulus, or developing stage."

10. D
The passage lists four ways that air is heated. One way is, heat created by water vapor condensing into liquid.

11. A
The sequence of events can be taken from these sentences:

As the moisture carried by the [1] air currents rises, it rapidly cools into liquid drops of water, which appear as cumulus clouds. As the water vapor condenses into liquid, it [2] releases heat, which warms the air. This in turn causes the air to become less dense than the surrounding dry air and [3] rise farther.

12. C
The purpose of this text is to explain when meteorologists consider a thunderstorm severe.

The main idea is the first sentence, "The United States National Weather Service classifies thunderstorms as severe when they reach a predetermined level." After the first sentence, the passage explains and elaborates on this idea. Everything is this passage is related to this idea, and there are no other major ideas in this passage that are central to the whole passage.

13. A
From this passage, we can infer that different areas and countries have different criteria for determining a severe storm.

From the passage we can see that most of the US has a criteria of, winds over 50 knots (58 mph or 93 km/h), and hail ¾ inch (2 cm). For the Central US, hail must be 1 inch (2.5 cm) in diameter. In Canada, winds must be 90 km/h or greater, hail 2 centimeters in diameter or greater, and rainfall more than 50 millimeters in 1 hour, or 75 millimeters in 3 hours.

Choice D is incorrect because the Canadian system is the same for hail, 2 centimeters in diameter.

14. C

With hail above the minimum size of 2.5 cm. diameter, the Central Region of the United States National Weather Service would issue a severe thunderstorm warning.

15. C

You would find information about natural selection and adaptation in the ecology section which begins on page 110.

16. D

Clouds in space are made of different materials attracted by gravity. Clouds on Earth are made of water droplets or ice crystals.

Choice D is the best answer. Notice also that Choice D is the most specific.

17. C

The main idea is the first sentence of the passage; a cloud is a visible mass of droplets or frozen crystals floating in the atmosphere above the surface of the Earth or other planetary body.

The main idea is very often the first sentence of the paragraph.

18. C

Nephology, which is the study of cloud physics.

19. C

This question asks about the process, and gives choices that can be confirmed or eliminated easily.

From the passage, "Dense, deep clouds reflect most light, so they appear white, at least from the top. Cloud droplets scatter light very efficiently, so the farther into a cloud light travels, the weaker it gets. This accounts for the gray or dark appearance at the base of large clouds."

We can eliminate choice A, since water droplets inside the cloud do not reflect light is false.

We can eliminate choice B, since, water droplets outside the cloud reflect light, it appears dark, is false.

Choice C is correct.

20. A
We know that an annex is like an attic because the text states the annex was above Otto Frank's building.

Option B is incorrect because an office building doesn't have bedrooms. Option C is incorrect because a basement would be below the office building. Option D is incorrect because there would not be a kitchen in an office building.

21. B
The diary has been published in 55 languages so people all over the world can learn about Anne. That is why the passage says it has been continuously in print.

Option A is incorrect because it is too vague. Option C is incorrect because it was published after Anne died and she did not write in all three languages. Option D is incorrect because the passage does not give us any information about what languages Otto Frank spoke.

22. C
Use the process of elimination to figure this out.

Option A cannot be the correct answer because otherwise the passage would have simply said that Anne and Margot both died of starvation. Options B and D cannot be correct because if the Germans had done something specifically to murder Anne, the passage would have stated that directly. By the process of elimination, Option C has to be the correct answer.

23. D
We can figure this out using context clues. The paragraph is talking about Anne's diary and so, outlet in this instance is a place where Anne can pour her feelings.

Option A is incorrect answer. That is the literal meaning of the word outlet and the passage is using the figurative meaning. Option B is incorrect because that is the secondary literal meaning of the word outlet, as in an outlet mall. Again, we are looking for figurative meaning. Option C is incorrect because there are no clues in the text to support that answer.

24. B
Reading the document posted to the Human Resources website is optional.

25. B
The document is recommended changes and have not be implemented yet.

26. A
Navy SEALs are the maritime component of the United States Special Operations Command (USSOCOM).

27. C
Working underwater separates SEALs from other military units. This is taken directly from the passage.

28. D
SEALs also belong to the Navy and the Coast Guard.

29. A
The CIA also participated. From the passage, the raid was conducted by a "team of 40 *CIA-led* Navy SEALs."

30. C
According to the blood pressure gauge, the patient's pulse is 62 beats per minute.

31. B
When someone is avid about something that means they are highly interested in the subject. The context clues are dull and boring, because they define the opposite of avid.

32. A
The author is using a simile to compare the books to medicine. Medicine is what you take when you want to feel better. They are suggesting that if a person wants to feel good, they

should read Dr. Seuss' books.

Option B is incorrect because there is no mention of a doctor's office. Option C is incorrect because it is using the literal meaning of medicine and the author is using medicine in a figurative way. Option D is incorrect because it makes no sense. We know not to eat books.

33. D
The publisher is described as intelligent because he knew to get in touch with a famous author to develop a book that children would be interested in reading.

Option A is incorrect because we can assume that all book publishers must know how to read. Option B is incorrect because it says in the article that more than one publisher was concerned about whether or not children liked to read. Option D is incorrect because there is no mention in the article about how well The Cat in the Hat sold when it was first published.

34. A
The Save the Children's fund has raised $12,000 out of $20,000, or 12/20. Simplifying, 12/20 = 3/5

35. B
The Save the Children's fund has raised $12,000 out of $16,000, or 12/16. Simplifying, 12/16 = 3/4

Section IV – Basic Science

1. A
Phenotype refers to observed properties of an organism and genotype refers to the genes of an organism.

2. A
A solution with a pH value of greater than 7 is a base.

3. A
Eukaryotic and prokaryotic cells are both organelles.

4. C
Homologous is being inherited by the organisms' common ancestors. An example would be feathers and hair—both of which were structures that shared a common ancestral trait.

5. C
The manner in which instructions for building proteins, the basic structural molecules of living material are written in the DNA is a genetic code.

6. C
A gene is a unit of inherited material, encoded by a strand of DNA and transcribed by RNA.

7. D
All of these statements are correct.

> a. During meiosis, the number of chromosomes in the cell are halved.
>
> b. Meiosis only occurs in eukaryotic cells.
>
> c. Meiosis is the part of the life cycle that involves sexual reproduction.

8. A Carrying capacity
An area's carrying capacity is the maximum number of animals of a given species that area can support during the harshest part of the year.

9. B
Diverticulitis is a pouch in the large intestine becomes inflamed.

10. A
Detection of pathogens can be complicated because they evolve so quickly.

11. A
Photosynthesis is the process by which plants and other photoautotrophs generate carbohydrates and oxygen from carbon dioxide, water, and light energy in chloroplasts.

12. C
Mutations in DNA sequences usually occur spontaneously is false.

Note: Mutations result when the DNA polymerase makes a mistake, which happens about once every 100,000,000 bases. Actually, the number of mistakes that remain incorporated into the DNA is even lower than this because cells contain special DNA repair proteins that fix many of the mistakes in the DNA that are caused by mutagens. The repair proteins see which nucleotides are paired incorrectly, and then change the wrong base to the right one. [14]

13. A
Starting with the weakest, the fundamental forces of nature in order of strength are, Gravity, Weak nuclear force, Electromagnetic force, Strong nuclear force.

Note: Although gravitational force is the weakest of the four, it acts over great distances. Electromagnetic force is of order 10^{39} times stronger than gravity.

14. A
Precision, which refers to the repeatability of measurement, does not require knowledge of the correct or true value.

15. A
Artificial selection is a process where desirable traits are systematically bred.

16. C
Condensation is not an example of vaporization. Boiling and evaporation are both examples of vaporization. Condensation is the process by which matter transitions from a gas to a liquid.

17. B
A periodic table is a tabular display of the chemical elements, organized on the basis of their atomic numbers, electron configurations, and recurring chemical properties.

18. A

In terms of the scientific method, the term observation refers to the act of noticing or perceiving something and/or recording a fact or occurrence.

19. B

Kinetic energy is the energy of a body that results from motion while potential energy is the energy possessed by an object by virtue of its position or state, e.g., as in a compressed spring.

20. A

A life cycle is the sequence of developmental stages through which members of a given species must pass.

21. A

The cell membrane is a biological membrane that separates the interior of all cells from the outside environment. The cell membrane is selectively permeable to ions and organic molecules and controls the movement of substances in and out of cells [6]

22. D

Relative position is not a taxonomic rank. Ranks include Domain, Kingdom, Phylum, Class, Order, Family, Genus, and Species.

23. D

The scientific term experiment refers to a practical test designed with the intention that its results be relevant to a particular theory or set of theories.

24. B

Substances that deactivate catalysts are called catalytic poisons.

25. B

Kinetic energy is the energy an object possesses due to its motion.

26. C
The interval of confidence around the measured value such
that the measured value is certain not to lie outside this
stated interval refers to the **uncertainty** of that value.

27. D
Arteries carry oxygenated blood away from the heart, veins
return oxygen-depleted blood to the heart, and capillaries
are thin-walled blood vessels in which gas/ nutrient/ waste
exchange occurs.

Note: An easy way to remember the difference between an
artery and a vein is that Arteries carry Away from the heart.

28. B
The thoracic diaphragm, or simply the diaphragm, is a sheet
of internal skeletal muscle that extends across the bottom
of the rib cage. The diaphragm separates the thoracic cavity
(heart, lungs & ribs) from the abdominal cavity and performs
an important function in respiration. [z]

29. D
Scientific classification. The two phrases are interchangeable, although the former seems to more accurately reflect
the purpose of classification: to categorize biological units.

30. C
A recessive gene is not expressed as a trait unless inherited
by both parents.

31. D
A scientific model is an approximation or simulation of a real
system that omits all but the most essential variables of the
system.

32. A
Neutrons are necessary within an atomic nucleus as they
bind with protons via the nuclear force.

33. C
The following statement is false - Most enzymes are inor-
ganic.

34. C
Acids are compounds that contain hydrogen and can dissolve in water to release hydrogen ions into solution.

35. A
Genes determine individual hereditary characteristics

36. A
The groups into which organisms are classified are called taxa and include, **in order of size**, Genus, Kingdom, Phylum/division, Class, Order, and Family Species.

37. D
Digestion begins in the mouth.

38. A
The main components of the circulatory system are the heart, veins and blood vessels.

39. D
An example of a pathogen that the immune system detects is a virus.

40. A
Chemical bonds are attractions between atoms that form chemical substances containing two or more atoms.

41. B
Cleansing food of impurities is not an example of a function of the stomach in digestion.

42. D
The exchange of oxygen for carbon dioxide takes place in the alveolar area of the lungs.

43. C
In chemistry, the number of protons in the nucleus of an atom is known as the atomic number, which determines the chemical element to which the atom belongs.

44. C
Natural selection is a process where biological traits become more or less common in a population

45. A
Females have two X chromosomes and males have one X chromosome and one Y chromosome.

46. A
The immune system fight off disease by identifying and killing tumor cells and pathogens.

47. A
Water has two hydrogen atoms covalently bonded to one oxygen atom

48. C
Choice C (Atomic theory explains temperature as the momentum of atoms.) is incorrect because atomic theory explains temperature as the motion of atoms (faster = hotter), not the momentum. The momentum of atoms explains the outward pressure that they exert.

49. D
Cardiac dysrhythmia (also known as arrhythmia and irregular heartbeat) is a term for any of a large and heterogeneous group of conditions in which there is abnormal electrical activity in the heart. The heart beat may be too fast or too slow, and may be regular or irregular. [8]

50. A
Eating a healthy diet is the best way to avoid most digestive diseases.

51. C
An important side-benefit of the respiratory system is the air being expelled from the mouth allows for speaking.

52. A
Emphysema is a long-term, progressive disease of the lungs that primarily causes shortness of breath. In people with emphysema, the tissues necessary to support the physical shape and function of the lungs are destroyed. It is included in a group of diseases called chronic obstructive pulmonary dis-

ease or COPD (pulmonary refers to the lungs). [19]

53. B
Inflammation is an example of an early response by the immune system to infection.
54. B
White blood cells are an important weapon in the fight against infection?

55. A
The complementary bases found in DNA are adenine and thymine or cytosine and guanine.

56. A
The term genome may be applied to the genetic information carried by an individual or to the range of genes found in a given species. The human genome is composed of 75,000 genes.

57. B
Taxonomy is a classification of organisms into different categories based on their physical characteristics and presumed natural relationship.

58. A
The order of the hierarchy of levels in the biological classification of organisms is: Kingdom, phylum, class, order, family, genus, and species.

59. A
A salt is any compound produced by a chemical reaction between a base and an acid.

60. A
A food web is a graphical description of feeding relationships among species in an ecological community.

Note: A food web differs from a food chain in that the latter shows only a portion of the food web involving a simple, linear series of species (e.g., predator, herbivore, plant) connected by feeding links. A food web aims to depict a more complete picture of the feeding relationships, and can be considered a bundle of many interconnected food chains occurring within the community.

Practice Test 2

Part 1 - Academic Aptitude

Verbal Sub-test – Vocabulary
Questions: 30
Time: 30 Minutes

Mathematics Sub-test
Questions: 30
Time: 30 Minutes

Nonverbal Sub-test
Questions: 30
Time: 30 Minutes

Part II – Spelling
Questions: 30
Time: 30 Minutes

Part III – Reading Comprehension
Questions: 35
Time: 35 Minutes

Part VI – Basic Science
Questions: 60
Time: 60 minutes

The practice test portion presents questions that are representative of the type of question you should expect to find on the PSB. However, they are not intended to match exactly what is on the PSB. Don't worry though! If you can answer these questions, you will have not trouble with the PSB.

For the best results, take this Practice Test as if it were the real exam. Set aside time when you will not be disturbed, and a location that is quiet and free of distractions. Read the instructions carefully, read each question carefully, and answer to the best of your ability.

Use the bubble answer sheets provided. When you have completed the Practice Test, check your answer against the Answer Key and read the explanation provided.

Part 1 – Vocabulary Sub-test

	A B C D E		A B C D E
1	○ ○ ○ ○ ○	21	○ ○ ○ ○ ○
2	○ ○ ○ ○ ○	22	○ ○ ○ ○ ○
3	○ ○ ○ ○ ○	23	○ ○ ○ ○ ○
4	○ ○ ○ ○ ○	24	○ ○ ○ ○ ○
5	○ ○ ○ ○ ○	25	○ ○ ○ ○ ○
6	○ ○ ○ ○ ○	26	○ ○ ○ ○ ○
7	○ ○ ○ ○ ○	27	○ ○ ○ ○ ○
8	○ ○ ○ ○ ○	28	○ ○ ○ ○ ○
9	○ ○ ○ ○ ○	29	○ ○ ○ ○ ○
10	○ ○ ○ ○ ○	30	○ ○ ○ ○ ○
11	○ ○ ○ ○ ○		
12	○ ○ ○ ○ ○		
13	○ ○ ○ ○ ○		
14	○ ○ ○ ○ ○		
15	○ ○ ○ ○ ○		
16	○ ○ ○ ○ ○		
17	○ ○ ○ ○ ○		
18	○ ○ ○ ○ ○		
19	○ ○ ○ ○ ○		
20	○ ○ ○ ○ ○		

Part II – Mathematics Sub-test

	A	B	C	D	E		A	B	C	D	E
1	○	○	○	○	○	21	○	○	○	○	○
2	○	○	○	○	○	22	○	○	○	○	○
3	○	○	○	○	○	23	○	○	○	○	○
4	○	○	○	○	○	24	○	○	○	○	○
5	○	○	○	○	○	25	○	○	○	○	○
6	○	○	○	○	○	26	○	○	○	○	○
7	○	○	○	○	○	27	○	○	○	○	○
8	○	○	○	○	○	28	○	○	○	○	○
9	○	○	○	○	○	29	○	○	○	○	○
10	○	○	○	○	○	30	○	○	○	○	○
11	○	○	○	○	○						
12	○	○	○	○	○						
13	○	○	○	○	○						
14	○	○	○	○	○						
15	○	○	○	○	○						
16	○	○	○	○	○						
17	○	○	○	○	○						
18	○	○	○	○	○						
19	○	○	○	○	○						
20	○	○	○	○	○						

Nonverbal Sub-test

	A	B	C	D	E		A	B	C	D	E
1	○	○	○	○	○	21	○	○	○	○	○
2	○	○	○	○	○	22	○	○	○	○	○
3	○	○	○	○	○	23	○	○	○	○	○
4	○	○	○	○	○	24	○	○	○	○	○
5	○	○	○	○	○	25	○	○	○	○	○
6	○	○	○	○	○	26	○	○	○	○	○
7	○	○	○	○	○	27	○	○	○	○	○
8	○	○	○	○	○	28	○	○	○	○	○
9	○	○	○	○	○	29	○	○	○	○	○
10	○	○	○	○	○	30	○	○	○	○	○
11	○	○	○	○	○						
12	○	○	○	○	○						
13	○	○	○	○	○						
14	○	○	○	○	○						
15	○	○	○	○	○						
16	○	○	○	○	○						
17	○	○	○	○	○						
18	○	○	○	○	○						
19	○	○	○	○	○						
20	○	○	○	○	○						

Part II – Spelling

	A	B	C	D	E		A	B	C	D	E
1	○	○	○	○	○	21	○	○	○	○	○
2	○	○	○	○	○	22	○	○	○	○	○
3	○	○	○	○	○	23	○	○	○	○	○
4	○	○	○	○	○	24	○	○	○	○	○
5	○	○	○	○	○	25	○	○	○	○	○
6	○	○	○	○	○	26	○	○	○	○	○
7	○	○	○	○	○	27	○	○	○	○	○
8	○	○	○	○	○	28	○	○	○	○	○
9	○	○	○	○	○	29	○	○	○	○	○
10	○	○	○	○	○	30	○	○	○	○	○
11	○	○	○	○	○						
12	○	○	○	○	○						
13	○	○	○	○	○						
14	○	○	○	○	○						
15	○	○	○	○	○						
16	○	○	○	○	○						
17	○	○	○	○	○						
18	○	○	○	○	○						
19	○	○	○	○	○						
20	○	○	○	○	○						

Part III – Reading Comprehension

	A	B	C	D	E		A	B	C	D	E
1	○	○	○	○	○	21	○	○	○	○	○
2	○	○	○	○	○	22	○	○	○	○	○
3	○	○	○	○	○	23	○	○	○	○	○
4	○	○	○	○	○	24	○	○	○	○	○
5	○	○	○	○	○	25	○	○	○	○	○
6	○	○	○	○	○	26	○	○	○	○	○
7	○	○	○	○	○	27	○	○	○	○	○
8	○	○	○	○	○	28	○	○	○	○	○
9	○	○	○	○	○	29	○	○	○	○	○
10	○	○	○	○	○	30	○	○	○	○	○
11	○	○	○	○	○	31	○	○	○	○	○
12	○	○	○	○	○	32	○	○	○	○	○
13	○	○	○	○	○	33	○	○	○	○	○
14	○	○	○	○	○	34	○	○	○	○	○
15	○	○	○	○	○	35	○	○	○	○	○
16	○	○	○	○	○						
17	○	○	○	○	○						
18	○	○	○	○	○						
19	○	○	○	○	○						
20	○	○	○	○	○						

Part IV - Natural Sciences

	A	B	C	D	E		A	B	C	D	E
1	○	○	○	○	○	31	○	○	○	○	○
2	○	○	○	○	○	32	○	○	○	○	○
3	○	○	○	○	○	33	○	○	○	○	○
4	○	○	○	○	○	34	○	○	○	○	○
5	○	○	○	○	○	35	○	○	○	○	○
6	○	○	○	○	○	36	○	○	○	○	○
7	○	○	○	○	○	37	○	○	○	○	○
8	○	○	○	○	○	38	○	○	○	○	○
9	○	○	○	○	○	39	○	○	○	○	○
10	○	○	○	○	○	40	○	○	○	○	○
11	○	○	○	○	○	41	○	○	○	○	○
12	○	○	○	○	○	42	○	○	○	○	○
13	○	○	○	○	○	43	○	○	○	○	○
14	○	○	○	○	○	44	○	○	○	○	○
15	○	○	○	○	○	45	○	○	○	○	○
16	○	○	○	○	○	46	○	○	○	○	○
17	○	○	○	○	○	47	○	○	○	○	○
18	○	○	○	○	○	48	○	○	○	○	○
19	○	○	○	○	○	49	○	○	○	○	○
20	○	○	○	○	○	50	○	○	○	○	○
21	○	○	○	○	○	51	○	○	○	○	○
22	○	○	○	○	○	52	○	○	○	○	○
23	○	○	○	○	○	53	○	○	○	○	○
24	○	○	○	○	○	54	○	○	○	○	○
25	○	○	○	○	○	55	○	○	○	○	○
26	○	○	○	○	○	56	○	○	○	○	○
27	○	○	○	○	○	57	○	○	○	○	○
28	○	○	○	○	○	58	○	○	○	○	○
29	○	○	○	○	○	59	○	○	○	○	○
30	○	○	○	○	○	60	○	○	○	○	○

Part 1 – Academic Aptitude - Vocabulary

1. a. Exigent b. Accurate c. Precise d. Undemanding

2. a. Inimical b. Amicable c. Friendly d. Sociable

3. a. Grapple b. Seize c. Prebend d. Unleash

4. a. Pervious b. Receptive c. Timorous d. Porous

5. a. Exorbitant b. Expensive c. Unconscionable d. Moderate

6. a. Unctuous b. Reprehensible c. Deplorable d. Vicious

7. a. Persuasive b. Admonitory c. Cautionary d. Exemplary

8. a. Talk b. Ponder c. Speak d. Pontificate

9. a. Address b. Speak c. Harangue d. Query

10. a. Adjourn b. Convoke c. Convene d. Summon

11. a. Decode b. Conform c. Decrypt d. Decipher

12. a. Discharge b. Exonerate c. Convict d. Exculpate

13. a. Elucidate b. Obfuscate c. Explain d. Explicate

14. a. Ardent b. Fervent c. Passionless d. Torrid

15. a. Taciturn b. Garrulous c. Loquacious d. Talkative

16. a. Intrepid b. Fearless c. Craven d. Brave

17. a. Jocular b. Amusing c. Uproarious d. Sober

18. a. Judicious b. Prudent c. Irrational d. Cautious

19. a. Lacerate b. Wound c. Rip d. Inculcate

20. a. Obligatory b. Elective c. Indispensable
d. Prerequisite

21. a. Obsolete b. Objectionable c. Obnoxious
d. Annoying

22. a. Rankle b. Grate c. Annoy d. Ingratiate

23. a. Verdure b. Greenness c. Freshness d. Expansive

24. a. Enthusiast b. Extremist c. Champion d. Zealot

25. a. Lithe b. Flexible c. Pliant d. Artificial

26. a. Pudgy b. Plump c. Overdone d. Fat

27. a. Aggravate b. Mollify c. Soothe d. Allay

28. a. Vex b. Assist c. Agitate d. Exasperate

29. a. Oblivious b. Abeyance c. Conscious d. Insensible

30. a. Abominate b. Abhor c. Cherish d. Loathe

Mathematics

1. Richard gives 's' amount of salary to each of his 'n' employees weekly. If he has 'x' amount of money then how many days he can employ these 'n' employees.

    a. sx/7n
    b. 7x/nx
    c. nx/7s
    d. 7x/ns

2. Translate the following into an equation: Five greater than 3 times a number.

    a. 3X + 5
    b. 5X + 3
    c. (5 + 3)X
    d. 5(3 + X)

3. What number is MMXIII?

    a. 2010

    b. 1990

    c. 2013

    d. 2012

4. It is known that $x^2+4x=5$. Then x can be

    a. 0

    b. -5

    c. 1

    d. Either (b) or (c)

5. Write 765.3682 to the nearest 1000th.

    a. 765.368

    b. 765.361

    c. 765.369

    d. 765.378

6. If Lynn can type a page in p minutes, what portion of the page can she do in 5 minutes?

    a. 5/p

    b. p - 5

    c. p + 5

    d. p/5

7. If Sally can paint a house in 4 hours, and John can paint the same house in 6 hours, how long will it take for both of them to paint the house together?

    a. 2 hours and 24 minutes

    b. 3 hours and 12 minutes

    c. 3 hours and 44 minutes

    d. 4 hours and 10 minutes

8. Employees of a discount appliance store receive an additional 20% off the lowest price on any item. If an employee purchases a dishwasher during a 15% off sale, how much will he pay if the dishwasher originally cost $450?

   a. $280.90

   b. $287

   c. $292.50

   d. $306

9. The sale price of a car is $12,590, which is 20% off the original price. What is the original price?

   a. $14,310.40

   b. $14,990.90

   c. $15,108.00

   d. $15,737.50

10. Express 25% as a fraction.

   a. 1/4

   b. 7/40

   c. 6/25

   d. 8/28

11. Express 125% as a decimal.

   a. .125

   b. 12.5

   c. 1.25

   d. 125

12. Express 24/56 as a reduced common fraction.

    a. 4/9

    b. 4/11

    c. 3/7

    d. 3/8

13. Express 71/1000 as a decimal.

    a. .71

    b. .0071

    c. .071

    d. 7.1

14. What number is in the ten thousandths place in 1.7389?

    a. 1

    b. 8

    c. 9

    d. 3

15. Simplify 6 3/5 – 4 4/5

    a. 2 4/5

    b. 2 3/5

    c. 2 9/5

    d. 1 1/5

16. The physician ordered 100 mg Ibuprofen/kg of body weight; on hand is 230 mg/tablet. The child weighs 50 lb. How many tablets will you give?

    a. 10 tablets

    b. 5 tablets

    c. 1 tablet

    d. 12 tablets

17. In a local election at polling station A, 945 voters cast their vote out of 1270 registered voters. At polling station B, 860 cast their vote out of 1050 registered voters and at station C, 1210 cast their vote out of 1440 registered voters. What is the total turnout including all three polling stations?

    a. 70%

    b. 74%

    c. 76%

    d. 80%

18. The physician ordered 600 mg ibuprofen. The office stocks 200 mg tablets. How many tablets will you give?

    a. 3.5 tablets

    b. 2 tablets

    c. 5 tablets

    d. 3 tablets

19. The manager of a weaving factory estimates that if 10 machines run on 100% efficiency for 8 hours, they will produce 1450 meters of cloth. However, due to some technical problems, 4 machines run of 95% efficiency and the remaining 6 at 90% efficiency. How many meters of cloth can these machines will produce in 8 hours?

    a. 1479 meters

    b. 1310 meters

    c. 1334 meters

    d. 1285 meters

20. Convert 60 feet to inches.

    a. 700 inches

    b. 600 inches

    c. 720 inches

    d. 1,800 inches

21. A box contains 7 black pencils and 28 blue ones. What is the ratio between the black and blue pens?

    a. 1:4

    b. 2:7

    c. 1:8

    d. 1:9

22. Convert 100 millimeters to centimeters.

    a. 10 centimeters

    b. 1,000 centimeters

    c. 1100 centimeters

    d. 50 centimeters

23. Convert 3 gallons to quarts.

    a. 15 quarts

    b. 6 quarts

    c. 12 quarts

    d. 32 quarts

24. A map uses a scale of 1:2,000 How much distance on the ground is 5.2 inches on the map if the scale is in inches?

    a. 100,400

    b. 10, 500

    c. 10,400

    d. 10,440

25. 0.05 ml. =

    a. 50 liters

    b. 0.00005 liters

    c. 5 liters

    d. 0.0005 liters

26. X% of 120 = 30. Solve for X.

    a. 15

    b. 12

    c. 4

    d. 25

27. Smith and Simon are playing a card game. Smith will win if a card drawn from a deck of 52 is either 7 or a diamond, and Simon will win if the drawn card is an even number. Which statement is more likely to be correct?

    a. Smith will win more games.

    b. Simon will win more games.

    c. They have same winning probability.

    d. A decision cannot be made from the provided data.

28. Convert .45 meters to centimeters

    a. 45

    b. 450

    c. 4.5

    d. .45

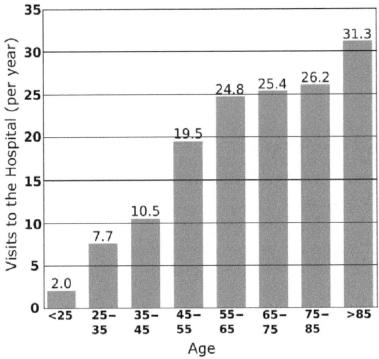

29. Consider the graph above.

How many hospital visits per year does a person aged 85 or more make?

    a. 26.2

    b. 31.3

    c. More than 31.3

    d. A decision cannot be made from this graph.

30. Based on this graph, how many visits per year do you expect a person that is 95 or older to make?

    a. More than 31.3

    b. Less than 31.3

    c. 31.3

    d. A decision cannot be made from this graph.

Nonverbal

1.

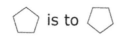 is to

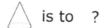 is to   ?

a. 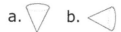   b.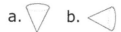

c. 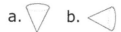   d.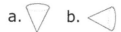

2.

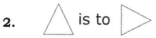 is to

 is to   ?

a. 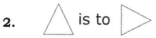   b.

c.   d.

3.

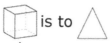 is to

is to   ?

a.   b.

c.   d.

4.

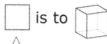 is to

is to   ?

a.   b.

c.   d.

5. ⬠ is to ⬡

⬡ is to ?

a. ☐   b. ⬡

c. ⬠   d. ⬡

6.

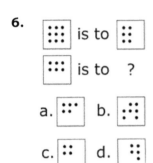

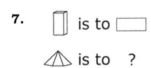

a. :::   b. :::

c. ::   d. ::

7. ▯ is to ▭

△ is to ?

a. ▷   b. ▭

c. ▷   d. ▢

8. ◯ is to ()

☐ is to ?

a. ▫   b. ▯

c. ▭   d. ▫

9. Winner : Champion :: Sheen :

   a. Shimmer

   b. Dark

   c. Sweet

   d. Garbage

10. Frog : Amphibian :: Snake :

   a. Reptile

   b. Protozoan

   c. Mammals

   d. Bacteria

11. Petal : Flower :: Fur

   a. Coat

   b. Warm

   c. Woman

   d. Rabbit

12. Present : Birthday :: Reward :

   a. Accomplishment

   b. Medal

   c. acceptance

   d. cash

13. Shovel : Dig :: Scissors :

   a. Scoop

   b. Carry

   c. Snip

   d. Rip

14. Finger : Hand :: Leg :

    a. Body

    b. Foot

    c. Toe

    d. Hip

15. Sleep in : Late :: Skip breakfast :

    a. Hungry

    b. Early

    c. Lunch

    d. Dinner

16. Circle : Sphere :: Square :

    a. Triangle

    b. Oval

    c. Half Circle

    d. Cube

17. Orange : Fruit :: Carrot:

    a. Vegetable

    b. Bean

    c. Food

    d. Apple

18. Which of the following does not belong?

    a. ddeeffgg

    b. ffgghhii

    c. nnooppqq

    d. ttuuvvww

19. **Which of the following does not belong?**

    a. 11223344
    b. 33445566
    c. 33455666
    d. 44556677

20. **Which of the following does not belong?**

    a. mNo
    b. pQr
    c. Stu
    d. xYz

21. **Which of the following does not belong?**

    a. abcabc
    b. defdef
    c. ghihij
    d. mnomno

22. **Which of the following does not belong?**

    a. Dog
    b. Wolf
    c. Terrier
    d. Cougar

23. **Which of the following does not belong?**

    a. DDDdddEEE
    b. MMMoooPPP
    c. GGGhhhIII
    d. JJJkkkLLL

24. Which of the following does not belong?

    a. cde

    b. mno

    c. stu

    d. abc

25. Which of the following does not belong?

    a. 446688

    b. 224466

    c. 336699

    d. 66881010

26. Which of the following does not belong?

    a. Assume

    b. Certain

    c. Sure

    d. Positive

27. Which of the following does not belong?

    a. MnOp

    b. AbCD

    c. QrSt

    d. WxYz

28. Which of the following does not belong?

    a. Look

    b. See

    c. Perceive

    d. Surmise

29. Which of the following does not belong?

    a. Count

    b. Number

    c. Add up

    d. List

30. Which of the following does not belong?

    a. Secure

    b. Discard

    c. Throw out

    d. Abandon

Part II – Spelling

1. Choose the correct spelling.

    a. corespondence

    b. corespodence

    c. correspodence

    d. correspomdence

2. Choose the correct spelling.

    a. henmorrhage

    b. hemmorrhage

    c. hemorrhage

    d. hemorhage

3. Choose the correct spelling.

    a. enviromnment

    b. environment

    c. environiment

    d. enviromment

4. Choose the correct spelling.

    a. govermment

    b. goverment

    c. govenment

    d. government

5. Choose the correct spelling.

    a. Conceeve

    b. Concieve

    c. Conceive

    d. Conceve

6. Choose the correct spelling.

    a. Describe

    b. Decribe

    c. Decsribe

    d. Discribe

7. Choose the correct spelling.

    a. Liqour

    b. Liquor

    c. Liquer

    d. Liquour

8. Choose the correct spelling.

    a. Succesful

    b. Sucessful

    c. Sucessfull

    d. Successful

9. Choose the correct spelling.

    a. Huricane

    b. Hurricane

    c. Huricane

    d. Hurriccane

10. Choose the correct spelling.

    a. Precede

    b. Preccede

    c. Precceed

    d. Preceed

11. Choose the correct spelling.

    a. Embarasment

    b. Embarrasment

    c. Imbarrassment

    d. Embarrassment

12. Choose the correct spelling.

    a. Cutastrophy

    b. Catastrophe

    c. Catastrophy

    d. Catustrophy

13. Choose the correct spelling.

    a. Hygeine

    b. Hygiene

    c. Hygene

    d. None of the Above

14. Choose the correct spelling.

    a. Embellish

    b. Embelish

    c. Imbelish

    d. Embillesh

15. Choose the correct spelling.

    a. Previlige

    b. Prevelige

    c. Privilege

    d. Privelige

16. Choose the correct spelling.

    a. Stupendos

    b. Stupendous

    c. Stupendouos

    d. Stupendues

17. Choose the correct spelling.

    a. Obletireate

    b. Obletirate

    c. Oblitterate

    d. Obliterate

18. Choose the correct spelling.

    a. Miscellaeneus

    b. Miscellaneous

    c. Micellaneous

    d. Miscellaneouos

19. Choose the correct spelling.

    a. Inoccuous

    b. Ennocuous

    c. Innoccuous

    d. Innocuous

20. Choose the correct spelling.

    a. Iminent

    b. Emminent

    c. Eminent

    d. Iminennt

21. Choose the correct spelling.

    a. Coalesque

    b. Coalesce

    c. Coalisque

    d. Coalisque

22. Choose the correct spelling.

    a. Bagage

    b. Buggage

    c. Baggage

    d. Bugage

23. Choose the correct spelling.

    a. Posible

    b. Possible

    c. Possibel

    d. None of the Above

24. Choose the correct spelling.

    a. Pronounce

    b. Prononce

    c. Pronunce

    d. Pronounse

25. Choose the correct spelling.

    a. Accesible

    b. Acessible

    c. Acesible

    d. Accessible

26. Choose the correct spelling.

    a. Idiosyncracy

    b. Idiosyncrassy

    c. Idiosyncrasy

    d. Idiocyncrasy

27. Choose the correct spelling.

    a. Kechup

    b. Ketsup

    c. Kechup

    d. Ketchup

28. Choose the correct spelling.

    a. Maintainance

    b. Maintenace

    c. Maintanance

    d. Maintenance

29. Choose the correct spelling.

    a. Humoros

    b. Humouros

    c. Humorous

    d. Humorus

30. Choose the correct spelling.

    a. Knowlege

    b. knowledge

    c. Knowlegde

    d. Knowlledge

Section 1 – Reading Comprehension

Questions 1-4 refer to the following passage.

Passage 1 - The Respiratory System

The respiratory system's function is to allow oxygen exchange through all parts of the body. The anatomy or structure of the exchange system, and the uses of the exchanged gases, varies depending on the organism. In humans and other mammals, for example, the anatomical features of the respiratory system include airways, lungs, and the respiratory muscles. Molecules of oxygen and carbon dioxide are passively exchanged, by diffusion, between the gaseous external environment and the blood. This exchange process occurs in the alveolar region of the lungs.

Other animals, such as insects, have respiratory systems with very simple anatomical features, and in amphibians even the skin plays a vital role in gas exchange. Plants also have respiratory systems but the direction of gas exchange can be opposite to that of animals.

The respiratory system can also be divided into physiological, or functional, zones. These include the conducting zone (the region for gas transport from the outside atmosphere to just above the alveoli), the transitional zone, and the respiratory zone (the alveolar region where gas exchange occurs). [11]

1. What can we infer from the first paragraph in this passage?

    a. Human and mammal respiratory systems are the same

    b. The lungs are an important part of the respiratory system

    c. The respiratory system varies in different mammals

    d. Oxygen and carbon dioxide are passive exchanged by the respiratory system

2. What is the process by which molecules of oxygen and carbon dioxide are passively exchanged?

    a. Transfusion

    b. Affusion

    c. Diffusion

    d. Respiratory confusion

3. What organ plays an important role in gas exchange in amphibians?

    a. The skin

    b. The lungs

    c. The gills

    d. The mouth

4. What are the three physiological zones of the respiratory system?

   a. Conducting, transitional, respiratory zones

   b. Redacting, transitional, circulatory zones

   c. Conducting, circulatory, inhibiting zones

   d. Transitional, inhibiting, conducting zones

Questions 5-8 refer to the following passage.

ABC Electric Warranty

ABC Electric Company warrants that its products are free from defects in material and workmanship. Subject to the conditions and limitations set forth below, ABC Electric will, at its option, either repair or replace any part of its products that prove defective due to improper workmanship or materials.

This limited warranty does not cover any damage to the product from improper installation, accident, abuse, misuse, natural disaster, insufficient or excessive electrical supply, abnormal mechanical or environmental conditions, or any unauthorized disassembly, repair, or modification.

This limited warranty also does not apply to any product on which the original identification information has been altered, or removed, has not been handled or packaged correctly, or has been sold as second-hand.

This limited warranty covers only repair, replacement, refund or credit for defective ABC Electric products, as provided above.

5. I tried to repair my ABC Electric blender, but could not, so can I get it repaired under this warranty?

    a. Yes, the warranty still covers the blender

    b. No, the warranty does not cover the blender

    c. Uncertain. ABC Electric may or may not cover repairs under this warranty

6. My ABC Electric fan is not working. Will ABC Electric provide a new one or repair this one?

    a. ABC Electric will repair my fan

    b. ABC Electric will replace my fan

    c. ABC Electric could either replace or repair my fan can request either a replacement or a repair.

7. My stove was damaged in a flood. Does this warranty cover my stove?

    a. Yes, it is covered.

    b. No, it is not covered.

    c. It may or may not be covered.

    d. ABC Electric will decide if it is covered

8. Which of the following is an example of improper workmanship?

    a. Missing parts

    b. Defective parts

    c. Scratches on the front

    d. None of the above

Questions 9 – 11 refer to the following passage.

Passage 2 – Mythology

The main characters in myths are usually gods or supernatural heroes. As sacred stories, rulers and priests have traditionally endorsed their myths and as a result, myths have a close link with religion and politics. In the society where a myth originates, the natives believe the myth is a true account of the remote past. In fact, many societies have two categories of traditional narrative—(1) "true stories," or myths, and (2) "false stories," or fables.

Myths generally take place during a primordial age, when the world was still young, prior to achieving its current form. These stories explain how the world gained its current form and why the culture developed its customs, institutions, and taboos. Closely related to myth are legend and folktale. Myths, legends, and folktales are different types of traditional stories. Unlike myths, folktales can take place at any time and any place, and the natives do not usually consider them true or sacred. Legends, on the other hand, are similar to myths in that many people have traditionally considered them true. Legends take place in a more recent time, when the world was much as it is today. In addition, legends generally feature humans as their main characters, whereas myths have superhuman characters. [12]

9. We can infer from this passage that

a. Folktales took place in a time far past, before civilization covered the earth

b. Humankind uses myth to explain how the world was created

c. Myths revolve around gods or supernatural beings; the local community usually accepts these stories as not true

d. The only difference between a myth and a legend is the time setting of the story

10. The main purpose of this passage is

a. To distinguish between many types of traditional stories, and explain the back-ground of some traditional story categories

b. To determine whether myths and legends might be true accounts of history

c. To show the importance of folktales how these traditional stories made life more bearable in harder times

d. None of the Above

11. How are folktales different from myths?

a.   Folktales and myth are the same

b.   Folktales are not true and generally not sacred and take place anytime

c.   Myths are not true and generally not sacred and take place anytime

d.   Folktales explained the formation of the world and myths do not

Getting Started

12. Based on the partial Table of Contents above, what is this book about?

a. How to answer multiple choice questions

b. Different types of multiple choice questions

c. How to write a test

d. None of the above

Questions 13-16 refer to the following passage.

Passage 3 – Myths, Legend and Folklore

Cultural historians draw a distinction between myth, legend and folktale simply as a way to group traditional stories. However, in many cultures, drawing a sharp line between myths and legends is not that simple. Instead of dividing their traditional stories into myths, legends, and folktales, some cultures divide them into two categories. The first category roughly corresponds to folktales, and the second is one that combines myths and legends. Similarly, we cannot always separate myths from folktales. One society might consider a story true, making it a myth. Another society may believe the story is fiction, which makes it a folktale. In fact, when a myth loses its status as part of a religious system, it often takes on traits more typical of folktales, with its formerly divine characters now appearing as human heroes, giants, or fairies. Myth, legend, and folktale are only a few of the categories of traditional stories. Other categories include anecdotes and some kinds of jokes. Traditional stories, in turn, are only one category within the larger category of folklore, which also includes items such as gestures, costumes, and music. [12]

13. The main idea of this passage is

a. Myths, fables, and folktales are not the same thing, and each describes a specific type of story

b. Traditional stories can be categorized in different ways by different people

c. Cultures use myths for religious purposes, and when this is no longer true, the people forget and discard these myths

d. Myths can never become folk tales, because one is true, and the other is false

14. The terms myth and legend are

a. Categories that are synonymous with true and false

b. Categories that group traditional stories according to certain characteristics

c. Interchangeable, because both terms mean a story that is passed down from generation to generation

d. Meant to distinguish between a story that involves a hero and a cultural message and a story meant only to entertain

15. Traditional story categories not only include myths and legends, but

a. Can also include gestures, since some cultures passed these down before the written and spoken word

b. In addition, folklore refers to stories involving fables and fairy tales

c. These story categories can also include folk music and traditional dress

d. Traditional stories themselves are a part of the larger category of folklore, which may also include costumes, gestures, and music

16. This passage shows that

a. There is a distinct difference between a myth and a legend, although both are folktales

b. Myths are folktales, but folktales are not myths

c. Myths, legends, and folktales play an important part in tradition and the past, and are a rich and colorful part of history

d. Most cultures consider myths to be true

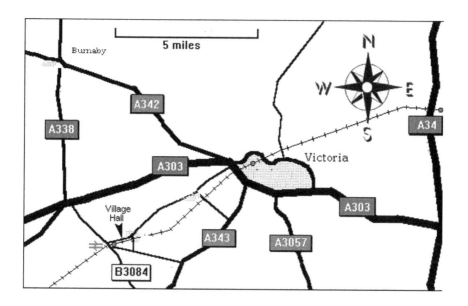

17. Approximately how far is Victoria to Burnaby?

a. About 10 miles

b. About 5 miles

c. About 15 miles

d. About 20 miles

18. How is the Village Hall from Victoria?

a. About 10 miles

b. About 5 miles

c. About 15 miles

d. About 20 miles

Questions 19 - 23 refer to the following passage.

Passage 4 – Trees I

Trees are an important part of the natural landscape because they prevent erosion and protect ecosystems in and under their branches. Trees also play an important role in producing oxygen and reducing carbon dioxide in the atmosphere, as well as moderating ground temperatures. Trees are important elements in landscaping and agriculture, both for their visual appeal and for their crops, such as apples, and other fruit. Wood from trees is a building material, and a primary energy source in many developing countries. Trees also play a role in many of the world's mythologies. [13]

19. What are two reasons trees are important in the natural landscape?

    a. They prevent erosion and produce oxygen

    b. They produce fruit and are important elements in landscaping

    c. Trees are not important in the natural landscape

    d. Trees produce carbon dioxide and prevent erosion

20. What kind of ecosystems do trees protect?

    a. Trees do not protect ecosystems

    b. Weather sheltered ecosystems

    c. Ecosystems around the base and under the branches

    d. All of the above

21. Which of the following is true?

   a. Trees provide a primary food source in the developing world

   b. Trees provide a primary building material in the developing world

   c. Trees provide a primary energy source in the developing world

   d. Trees provide a primary oxygen source in the developing world

22. Why are trees important for agriculture?

   a. Because of their crops

   b. Because they shelter ecosystems

   c. Because they are a source of energy

   d. Because of their visual appeal

23. What do trees do to the atmosphere?

   a. Trees produce carbon dioxide and reduce oxygen

   b. Trees product oxygen and carbon dioxide

   c. Trees reduce oxygen and carbon dioxide

   d. Trees produce oxygen and reduce carbon dioxide

Questions 24 - 27 refer to the following passage.

Passage 5 – The Life of Helen Keller

Many people have heard of Helen Keller. She is famous because she was unable to see or hear, but learned to speak and read and went onto attend college and earn a degree. Her life is a very interesting story, one that she developed into an autobiography, which was then adapted into both a stage play and a movie. How did Helen Keller overcome her disabilities to become a famous woman? Read onto find out.

Helen Keller was not born blind and deaf. When she was a small baby, she had a very high fever for several days. As a result of her sudden illness, baby Helen lost her eyesight and her hearing. Because she was so young when she went deaf and blind, Helen Keller never had any recollection of being able to see or hear. Since she could not hear, she could not learn to talk. Since she could not see, it was difficult for her to move around. For the first six years of her life, her world was very still and dark.

Imagine what Helen's childhood must have been like. She could not hear her mother's voice. She could not see the beauty of her parent's farm. She could not recognize who was giving her a hug, or a bath or even where her bedroom was each night. More sad, she could not communicate with her parents in any way. She could not express her feelings or tell them the things she wanted. It must have been a very sad childhood.

When Helen was six years old, her parents hired her a teacher named Anne Sullivan. Anne was a young woman who was almost blind. However, she could hear and she could read Braille, so she was a perfect teacher for young Helen. At first, Anne had a very hard time teaching Helen anything. She described her first impression of Helen as a "wild thing, not a child." Helen did not like Anne at first either. She bit and hit Anne when Anne tried to teach her. However, the two of them eventually came to have a great deal of love and respect.

Anne taught Helen to hear by putting her hands on people's throats. She could feel the sounds that people made. In time, Helen learned to feel what people said. Next, Anne taught Helen to read Braille, which is a way that books are written for the blind. Finally, Anne taught Helen to talk. Although Helen did learn to talk, it was hard for anyone but Anne to understand her.

As Helen grew older, more and more people were amazed by her story. She went to college and wrote books about her life. She gave talks to the public, with Anne at her side, translating her words. Today, both Anne Sullivan and Helen Keller are famous women who are respected for their lives' work.

24. Helen Keller could not see and hear and so, what was her biggest problem in childhood?

    a. Inability to communicate

    b. Inability to walk

    c. Inability to play

    d. Inability to eat

25. Helen learned to hear by feeling the vibrations people made when they spoke. What were these vibrations were felt through?

    a. Mouth

    b. Throat

    c. Ears

    d. Lips

26. From the passage, we can infer that Anne Sullivan was a patient teacher. We can infer this because

    a. Helen hit and bit her and Anne still remained her teacher.

    b. Anne taught Helen to read only.

    c. Anne was hard of hearing too.

    d. Anne wanted to be a teacher.

27. Helen Keller learned to speak but Anne translated her words when she spoke in public. The reason Helen needed a translator was because

    a. Helen spoke another language.

    b. Helen's words were hard for people to understand.

    c. Helen spoke very quietly.

    d. Helen did not speak but only used sign language.

Questions 28 - 30 refer to the following passage.

Lowest Price Guarantee

Get it for less. Guaranteed!

ABC Electric will beat any advertised price by 10% of the difference.

> 1) If you find a lower advertised price, we will beat it by 10% of the difference.
>
> 2) If you find a lower advertised price within 30 days* of your purchase we will beat it by 10% of the difference.
>
> 3) If our own price is reduced within 30 days* of your purchase, bring in your receipt and we will refund the difference.

*14 days for computers, monitors, printers, laptops, tablets, cellular & wireless devices, home security products, projectors, camcorders, digital cameras, radar detectors, portable DVD players, DJ and pro-audio equipment, and air conditioners.

28. I bought a radar detector 15 days ago and saw an ad for the same model only cheaper. Can I get 10% of the difference refunded?

> a. Yes. Since it is less than 30 days, you can get 10% of the difference refunded.
>
> b. No. Since it is more than 14 days, you cannot get 10% of the difference re-funded.
>
> c. It depends on the cashier.
>
> d. Yes. You can get the difference refunded.

29. I bought a flat-screen TV for $500 10 days ago and found an advertisement for the same TV, at another store, on sale for $400. How much will ABC refund under this guarantee?

    a. $100

    b. $110

    c. $10

    d. $400

30. What is the purpose of this passage?

    a. To inform

    b. To educate

    c. To persuade

    d. To entertain

Questions 31 - 33 refer to the following passage.

Passage 6 - What Is Mardi Gras?

Mardi Gras is fast becoming one of the South's most famous and most celebrated holidays. The word Mardi Gras comes from the French and the literal translation is "Fat Tuesday." The holiday has also been called Shrove Tuesday, due to its associations with Lent. The purpose of Mardi Gras is to celebrate and enjoy before the Lenten season of fasting and repentance begins.

What originated by the French Explorers in New Orleans, Louisiana in the 17th century is now celebrated all over the world. Panama, Italy, Belgium and Brazil all host large scale Mardi Gras celebrations, and many smaller cities and towns celebrate this fun loving Tuesday as well. Usually held in February or early March, Mardi Gras is a day of extravagance, a day for people to eat, drink and be merry, to wear costumes, masks and to dance to jazz music.
The French explorers on the Mississippi River would be in shock today if they saw the opulence of the parades and

floats that grace the New Orleans streets during Mardi Gras these days. Parades in New Orleans are divided by organizations. These are more commonly known as Krewes.

Being a member of a Krewe is quite a task because Krewes are responsible for overseeing the parades. Each Krewe's parade is ruled by a Mardi Gras "King and Queen." The role of the King and Queen is to "bestow" gifts on their adoring fans as the floats ride along the street. They throw doubloons, which is fake money and usually colored green, purple and gold, which are the colors of Mardi Gras. Beads in those color shades are also thrown and cups are thrown as well. Beads are by far the most popular souvenir of any Mardi Gras parade, with each spectator attempting to gather as many as possible.

31. The purpose of Mardi Gras is to

  a. Repent for a month.

  b. Celebrate in extravagant ways.

  c. Be a member of a Krewe.

  d. Explore the Mississippi.

32. From reading the passage we can infer that "Kings and Queens"

  a. Have to be members of a Krewe.

  b. Have to be French.

  c. Have to know how to speak French.

  d. Have to give away their own money.

33. Which group of people first began to hold Mardi Gras celebrations?

  a. Settlers from Italy

  b. Members of Krewes

  c. French explorers

  d. Belgium explorers

Questions 33-35 refer to the following passage.

Passage 7 - The Circulatory System

The circulatory system is an organ system that passes nutrients (such as amino acids and electrolytes), gases, hormones, and blood cells to and from cells in the body to help fight diseases and help stabilize body temperature and pH levels.

The circulatory system may be seen strictly as a blood distribution network, but some consider the circulatory system as composed of the cardiovascular system, which distributes blood, and the lymphatic system, which distributes lymph. While humans, as well as other vertebrates, have a closed cardiovascular system (meaning that the blood never leaves the network of arteries, veins and capillaries), some invertebrate groups have an open cardiovascular system. The most primitive animal phyla lack circulatory systems. The lymphatic system, on the other hand, is an open system.

Two types of fluids move through the circulatory system: blood and lymph. The blood, heart, and blood vessels form the cardiovascular system. The lymph, lymph nodes, and lymph vessels form the lymphatic system. The cardiovascular system and the lymphatic system collectively make up the circulatory system.

The main components of the human cardiovascular system are the heart and the blood vessels. It includes: the pulmonary circulation, a "loop" through the lungs where blood is oxygenated; and the systemic circulation, a "loop" through the rest of the body to provide oxygenated blood. An average adult contains five to six quarts (roughly 4.7 to 5.7 liters) of blood, which consists of plasma, red blood cells, white blood cells, and platelets. Also, the digestive system works with the circulatory system to provide the nutrients the system needs to keep the heart pumping. [14]

33. What can we infer from the first paragraph?

a. An important purpose of the circulatory system is that of fighting diseases.

b. The most important function of the circulatory system is to give the person energy.

c. The least important function of the circulatory system is that of growing skin cells.

d. The entire purpose of the circulatory system is not known.

34. Do humans have an open or closed circulatory system?

a. Open

b. Closed

c. Usually open, though sometimes closed

d. Usually closed, though sometimes open

35. In addition to blood, what two components form the cardiovascular system?

a. The heart and the lungs

b. The lungs and the veins

c. The heart and the blood vessels

d. The blood vessels and the nerves

Section IV – Basic Science

1. Which of the following is not true:

a. Genotypes are inherited information

b. Phenotypes are inherited information

c. Phenotypes are observed behavior

d. Phenotypes include an organisms development

2. Electrons play a critical role in:

a. Electricity

b. Magnetism

c. Thermal conductivity

d. All of the above

3. An idea concerning a phenomena and possible explanations for that phenomena is a/an

a. Theory

b. Experiment

c. Inference

d. Hypothesis

4. Define chromosomes.

a. Structures in a cell nucleus that carry genetic material.

b. Consist of thousands of DNA strands.

c. Total 46 in a normal human cell.

d. all of the above

5. What is one of the best known disorders that attack the immune system?

a. Rabies

b. HIV

c. Lung cancer

d. Muscular dystrophy

6. Which disease of the circulatory system is one of the most frequent causes of death in North America?

    a. The cold

    b. Pneumonia

    c. Arthritis

    d. Heart disease

7. Which of the following describes a plasma membrane?

    a. Lipids with embedded proteins

    b. An outer lipid layer and an inner lipid layer

    c. Proteins embedded in lipid bilayer

    d. Altering protein and lipid layers

8. What is the difference between Strong Nuclear Force and Weak Nuclear Force?

    a. The Strong Nuclear Force is an attractive force that binds protons and neutrons and maintains the structure of the nucleus, and the Weak Nuclear Force is responsible for the radioactive beta decay and other subatomic reactions.

    b. The Strong Nuclear Force is responsible for the radioactive beta decay and other subatomic reactions, and the Weak Nuclear Force is an attractive force that binds protons and neutrons and maintains the structure of the nucleus.

    c. The Weak Nuclear Force is feeble and the Strong Nuclear Force is robust.

    d. The Strong Nuclear Force is a negative force that releases protons and neutrons and threatens the structure of the nucleus, and the Weak Nuclear Force is an attractive force that binds protons and neutrons and maintains the structure of the nucleus.

9. What type of research deals with the quality, type or components of a group, substance, or mixture.

a. Quantitative

b. Dependent

c. Scientific

d. Qualitative

10. Adaptation is:

a. A trait that has evolved by natural selection

b. A trait that has been bred by artificial selection

c. A trait that has no function in an organism

d. None of the above

11. Describe a pH indicator.

a. A pH indicator measures hydrogen ions in a solution and show pH on a color scale.

b. A pH indicator measures oxygen ions in a solution and show pH on a color scale.

c. A pH indicator many different types of ions in a solution and shows pH on a color scale

d. None of the above

12. What is the earth's primary source of energy?

a. Water

b. The sun

c. Electromagnetic radiation

d. Weak nuclear force

13. What type of research is to determine the relationship between one thing (an independent variable) and another (a dependent or outcome variable) in a population.

    a. Qualitative

    b. Quantitative

    c. Independent

    d. Scientific

14. What can accept a hydrogen ion and can react with fats to form soaps?

    a. Acid

    b. Salt

    c. Base

    d. Foundation

15. Which gene, whose presence as a single copy, controls the expression of a trait?

    a. Principal gene

    b. Latent gene

    c. Recessive gene

    d. Dominant gene

16. Within taxonomy, plants and animals are considered two basic _____.

    a. Families

    b. Kingdoms

    c. Domains

    d. Genus

17. Organisms grouped into the _____ Kingdom include all unicellular organisms lacking a definite cellular arrangement such as _____ and _____.

    a. Fungi, bacteria, algae

    b. Protista, bacteria, amphibian

    c. Protista, bacteria, algae

    d. Plantae, bacteria, algae

18. What is a common digestive affliction that most people suffer at one time or other?

    a. Stomach cancer

    b. Ulceritis

    c. Indigestion

    d. The flu

19. What are the biochemical and biophysical activities that all living systems must be able to carry out to maintain life?

    a. Life sequences

    b. Life expectancies

    c. Life cycles

    d. Life functions

20. What disease of the circulatory system is often mistaken for a heart attack?

    a. Cardiac arrest

    b. High blood pressure

    c. Angina

    d. Acid reflux

21. Define a biological class.

    a. A collection of similar or like living entities.

    b. Two or more animals in a group, all having the same parent.

    c. All animals sharing the same living environment.

    d. All plant life that share the same physical properties.

22. What type of foods that stay in the stomach longest?

    a. Fats

    b. Proteins

    c. Carbohydrates

    d. Vitamins

23. How many elements are represented on the periodic table?

    a. 122 elements

    b. 99 elements

    c. 102 elements

    d. 118 elements

24. What is the diagram that is used to predict an outcome of a particular cross or breeding experiment?

    a. Genetic puzzle

    b. Genome project

    c. Hybrid theorem

    d. Punnett square

25. Which, if any, of the following statements about prokaryotic cells is false?

a. Prokaryotic cells include such organisms as E. coli and Streptococcus.

b. Prokaryotic cells lack internal membranes and organelles.

c. Prokaryotic cells break down food using cellular respiration and fermentation.

d. All of these statements are true.

26. What is the process of converting observed phenomena into data is called?

a. Calculation

b. Measurement

c. Valuation

d. Estimation

27. The mass number of an atom is:

a. The total number of particles that make it up

b. The total weight of an atom

c. The total mass of an atom

d. None of the above

28. What is sublimation?

a. A phase transition from liquid to gas

b. A phase transition from solid to gas

c. A phase transition from gas to liquid

d. A phase transition from gas to solid

29. How is exhalation accomplished?

a. By the abdominal muscles

b. By the chest muscles

c. By the esophagus

d. By the nasal passageway

30. What three processes are involved in cell division of Eukaryotic cells?

a. Meiosis, cytokinesis, and interphase

b. Meiosis, mitosis, and interphase

c. Mitosis, kinematisis, and interphase

d. Mitosis, cytokinesis, and interphase

31. Describe genotypes.

a. The genetic makeup, as distinguished from the physical appearance, of an organism or a group of organisms.

b. The combination of alleles located on homologous chromosomes that determines a specific characteristic or trait.

c. Is the inheritable information carried by all living organisms.

d. All of the above.

32. What does the respiratory system primarily oxygenate?

a. The brain

b. The limbs

c. The heart

d. The blood

33. What chain of nucleotides plays an important role in the creation of new proteins?

a. Deoxyribonucleic acid (DNA) is a chain of nucleotides that plays an important role in the creation of new proteins.

b. Ribonucleic acid (RNA) is a chain of nucleotides that plays an important role in the creation of new proteins.

c. There are no chains of nucleotides that play a role in the creation of proteins.

d. None of the above.

34. A practical test designed with the intention that its results will be relevant to a particular theory or set of theories is a/an

a. Experiment

b. Practicum

c. Theory

d. Design

35. Strong chemical bonds include

a. Dipole - dipole interactions

b. Hydrogen bonding

c. Covalent or ionic bonds

d. None of the above

36. What is the process that the immune system adapts over time to be more efficient in recognizing pathogens?

a. Acquired immunity

b. AIDS

c. Pathogens

d. Acquired deficiency

37. What is a group of tissues that perform a specific function or group of functions?

a. System

b. Tissue

c. Group

d. Organ

38. What is the measure of an experiment's ability to yield the same or compatible results in different clinical experiments or statistical trials?

a. Variability

b. Validity

c. Control measure

d. Reliability

39. Describe each chemical element in the periodic table.

a. Each chemical element has a unique atomic number representing the number of electrons in its nucleus.

b. Each chemical element has a varying atomic number depending on the number of protons in its nucleus.

c. Each chemical element has a unique atomic number representing the number of protons in its nucleus.

d. None of the above.

40. The immune system is

a. The system that expels waste from the body.

b. The system that expels carbon dioxide from the body.

c. The system that protects the body from disease and infection.

d. The system that circulates blood through the body.

41. The binding membrane of an animal cell is called

a. The biological membrane

b. The cell coat

c. The unit membrane

d. The plasma membrane

42. Define organelles

a. A protein in a cell

b. An enzyme in a cell

c. A specialized subunit of a cell with a specific function

d. A cell membrane

43. A solution with a pH value of less than 7 is

a. Acid solution

b. Base solution

c. Neutral pH solution

d. None of the above

44. Is a catalyst changed by a reaction?

a. Yes

b. No

c. It may be changed depending on the other chemicals

45. The _____ is the prediction that an observed difference is due to chance alone and not due to a systematic cause; this hypothesis is tested by statistical analysis, and either accepted or rejected.

a. Null hypothesis

b. Hypothesis

c. Control

d. Variable

46. In science, industry, and statistics, the _____ of a measurement system is the degree of closeness of measurements of a quantity to its actual (true) value.

    a. Mistake

    b. Uncertainty

    c. Accuracy

    d. Error

47. What is a more common name for the circulatory system disease known as hypertension?

    a. Anemia

    b. High blood pressure

    c. Angina

    d. Cardiac arrest

48. The ____ of a distribution is the difference between the maximum value and the minimum value.

    a. Distribution

    b. Range

    c. Mode

    d. Median

49. What is a statistical technique which determines if two variables are related.

    a. Statistical correlation

    b. Statistical measurement

    c. Control group

    d. Statistical analysis

50. What is the mathematical average of a set of numbers.

   a. Mean

   b. Median

   c. Distribution

   d. Standard deviation

51. What is the simplest unit of any compound?

   a. Atom

   b. Proton

   c. Molecule

   d. Compound

52. What results when acid reacts with a base?

   a. A weak acid

   b. A weak base

   c. A salt and water

   d. Hydrogen

53. The horizontal rows of the periodic table are known as

   a. Groups

   b. Periods

   c. Series

   d. Columns

54. When do oxidation and reduction reactions occur?

   a. One after the other

   b. In separate reactions

   c. On the product side of the reaction

   d. Simultaneously

55. What are most of the elements on the periodic table classified as?

    a. Nonmetals

    b. Metals

    c. Metalloids

    d. Gases

56. What is usually the result when acid reacts with most of the metals?

    a. Carbon dioxide

    b. Oxygen gas

    c. Nitrogen gas

    d. Hydrogen gas

57. What are the vertical columns of the periodic table?

    a. Series

    b. Groups

    c. Periods

    d. Columns

58. In a redox reaction, how many electrons are lost?

    a. Less than the number of electrons gained

    b. More than the number of electrons gained

    c. Equal to the number of electrons gained

    d. None of the above

59. A substance containing atoms of more than one element in a definite ratio is called a(n)

    a. Compound

    b. Element

    c. Mixture

    d. Molecule

60. All acids turn blue litmus paper

a. Blue

b. Red

c. Green

d. White

Answer Key

Part 1 Academic Aptitude

Vocabulary

1. D
2. A
3. D
4. C
5. D
6. A
7. A
8. B
9. D
10. A
11. B
12. C
13. B
14. C
15. A
16. C
17. D
18. C
19. D
20. B
21. A
22. D
23. D
24. C
25. D
26. C
27. A
28. B
29. C
30. C

Mathematics

1. D
We understand that each of the n employees earn s amount of salary weekly. This means that one employee earns s salary

weekly. So; Richard has ns amount of money to employ n employees for a week.

We are asked to find the number of days n employees can be employed with x amount of money. We can do simple direct proportion:

If Richard can employ n employees for 7 days with ns amount of money,

Richard can employ n employees for y days with x amount of money ... y is the number of days we need to find.

We can do cross multiplication:

$y = (x \cdot 7)/(ns)$

$y = 7x/ns$

2. A
Five greater than 3 times a number.
5 + 3 times a number.
$3X + 5$

3. C
MMXIII is 2013. 1,000 + 1,000 + 10 + 1 + 1 + 1.

4. D
$x2 + 4x = 5$, $x2 + 4x - 5 = 0$, $x2 + 5x - x - 5 = 0$, factorize $x(x + 5) -1(x + 5) = o$, $(x + 5)(x - 1) = 0$. $x + 5 = 0$ or $x - 1 = 0$, $x = 0 - 5$ or $x = 0 + 1$, $x = -5$ or $x = 1$, either b or c.

5. A
The number is 51.738. The last digit, in the 1,000th place, 2, is less than 5, so it is discarded. Answer = 765.368.

6. D
This is a simple direct proportion problem:
If Lynn can type 1 page in p minutes,

 she can type x pages in 5 minutes

We do cross multiplication: x•p = 5•1

Then,

x = 5/p

7. A
This is an inverse ration problem.

1/x = 1/a + 1/b where a is the time Sally can paint a house, b is the time John can paint a house, x is the time Sally and John can together paint a house.

So,

1/x = 1/4 + 1/6 ... We use the least common multiple in the denominator that is 24:

1/x = 6/24 + 4/24

1/x = 10/24

x = 24/10

x = 2.4 hours.

In other words; 2 hours + 0.4 hours = 2 hours + 0.4•60 minutes

= 2 hours 24 minutes

8. D
The cost of the dishwasher = $450

15% discount amount = 450•15/100 = $67.5

The discounted price = 450 – 67.5 = $382.5

20% additional discount amount on lowest price = 382.5•20/100 = $76.5

So, the final discounted price = 382.5 - 76.5 = $306.00

9. D
Original price = x,
80/100 = 12590/X,
80X = 1259000,
X = 15,737.50.

10. A
25% = 25/100 = 1/4

11. C
125/100 = 1.25

12. C
24/56 = 3/7 (divide numerator and denominator by 8)

13. C
Converting a fraction into a decimal – divide the numerator
by the denominator – so 71/1000 = .071. Dividing by 1000
moves the decimal point 3 places to the left.

14. C
9 is in the ten thousandths place in 1.7389, which is 4
places to the right of the decimal point.

15. A
(6-4) (3/5 – 4/5) = 2 (3-4/5) = since 3 is less than 4, we
would have to subtract 1 from the whole number besides the
fraction, therefore 1 13-4/5 = 1 9/5 = 2 4/5

16. A
Step 1: Set up the formula to calculate the dose to be given
in mg as per weight of the child:-
Dose ordered X Weight in Kg = Dose to be given
Step 2: 100 mg X 23 kg = 2300 mg
(Convert 50 lb to Kg, 1 lb = 0.4536 kg, hence 50 lb = 50 X
0.4536 = 22.68 kg
approx. 23 kg)
2300 mg/230 mg X 1 tablet/1 = 2300/230 = 10 tablets

17. D
To find the total turnout in all three polling stations, we
need to proportion the number of voters to the number of all

registered voters.

Number of total voters = 945 + 860 + 1210 = 3015

Number of total registered voters = 1270 + 1050 + 1440 = 3760

Percentage turnout over all three polling stations = 3015•100/3760 = 80.19%

Checking the answers, we round 80.19 to the nearest whole number: 80%

18. D
600 mg/ 200 mg X 1 tablet/1 = 600/200 = 3 tablets

19. C
At 100% efficiency 1 machine produces 1450/10 = 145 m of cloth.

At 95% efficiency, 4 machines produce 4•145•95/100 = 551 m of cloth.

At 90% efficiency, 6 machines produce 6•145•90/100 = 783 m of cloth.

Total cloth produced by all 10 machines = 551 + 783 = 1334 m

Since the information provided and the question are based on 8 hours, we did not need to use time to reach the answer.

20. C
1 foot = 12 inches, 60 feet = 60 x 12 = 720 inches.

21. A
The ratio between black and blue pens is 7 to 28 or 7:28. Bring to the lowest terms by dividing both sides by 7 gives 1:4.

22. A
1 millimeter = 10 centimeter, 100 millimeter = 100/10 = 10 centimeters.

23. C
1 gallon = 4 quarts, 3 gallons = 3 x 4 = 12 quarts.

24. D
1 inch on map = 2,000 inches on ground. So, 5.2 inches on map = 5.2•2,000 = 10,400 inches on ground.

25. B
There are 1000 ml in a liter. 0.05/1000 = 0.00005 liters.

26. D
X% of 120 = 30,
X/100 = 10/120
so X = 30/120 x 100/1
3000/120 = 300/12
X = 25

27. B
There are 52 cards in total. Smith has 16 cards in which he can win. Therefore, his probability of winning in a single game will be 16/52. Simon has 20 winning cards so his probability of winning in single draw is 20/52.

28. A
There are 100 centimeters in a meter, so 100 X .45 meters = 45 centimeters.

29. A
Based on this graph, a person that is 85 will make 26.2 visits to the hospital every year.

30. C
A person aged 95 or older would make more than 31.3 visits.

Nonverbal

1. A
The relation is the same figure rotated.

2. D
The relation is the same figure rotated.

3. B
The relation is a 3-dimensional figure to a 2-dimensional figure.

4. B
The relation is a 2-dimensional figure to a 3-dimensional figure.

5. B
The relation is a n-sided figure to an n+1 sided figure.

6. C
The first figure has 9 cots in a square and the second figure has 6 dots, which is 1/3 removed.

7. C
The relation is a 3-dimentional figure to a rotated 2-dimentional figure.

8. C
The relation is the same figure with the bottom half removed.

9. A
This is a synonym relationship. Shimmer has the same meaning as sheen.

10. A
This is a classification relationship. Reptile is the classification taxa for snake.

11. D
This is a part-to-whole relationship. A petal is to a flower as fur is to a rabbit.

12. A
A present celebrates a birthday and a reward celebrates an accomplishment.

13. C
This is a functional relationship. A shovel is used to dig and scissors are used to snip.

14. A

This is a parts-to-whole relationship. The finger is part of the hand in the same way a leg is part of a body.

15. A

This is a cause and effect relationship. If you sleep in you will be late. If you skip breakfast, you will be hungry.

16. D

A sphere is the solid form of a circle just as a cube is the solid form of a square.

17. A

This is a classification relationship. An orange is a fruit and a carrot is a vegetable.

18. B

This is a vowel and consonant relationship. All the choices have vowels in positions 3 and 4.

19. C

This is a repetition pattern. All the choices have consecutive numbers repeated twice.

20. C

This is a capital to small letter relationship. All choices have the middle letter capitalized.

21. C

This is a repetition pattern. All the choices repeat a three number sequence.

22. D

This is a relationship of words question. All the choices are dog or canine family except cougar.

23. B

This is a repetition pattern. All the choices repeat consecutive 3-number patterns.

24. D

This is a vowel and consonant relationship. All the choices have a vowel at the end.

25. C
This is a repetition pattern. All the choices repeat a 2-letter sequence obtained by adding two to the previous number.

26. A
This is a word meaning relationship. Assume is not a synonym for any of the choices.

27. B
This is a capital small letter relationship. All choices have alternate letters capitalized.

28. D
This is a relationship of words question. All the choices are synonyms of look and see, except surmise.

29. D
This is a word meaning relationship. List is not a synonym for any of the choices.

30. A
All of choices are synonyms of discard except secure.

Part II – Spelling

1. A
2. C
3. B
4. D
5. C
6. A
7. B
8. D
9. B
10. A
11. D
12. B
13. B
14. A
15. C
16. B
17. D

18. **B**
19. **D**
20. **C**
21. **B**
22. **C**
23. **B**
24. **A**
25. **D**
26. **C**
27. **D**
28. **D**
29. **C**
30. **B**

Part III Reading Comprehension

1. B

We can infer an important part of the respiratory system are the lungs. From the passage, "Molecules of oxygen and carbon dioxide are passively exchanged, by diffusion, between the gaseous external environment and the blood. This exchange process occurs in the alveolar region of the lungs."

Therefore, one of the primary functions for the respiratory system is the exchange of oxygen and carbon dioxide, and this process occurs in the lungs. We can therefore infer that the lungs are an important part of the respiratory system.

2. C

The process by which molecules of oxygen and carbon dioxide are passively exchanged is diffusion.

This is a definition type question. Scan the passage for references to "oxygen," "carbon dioxide," or "exchanged."

3. A

The organ that plays an important role in gas exchange in amphibians is the skin.

Scan the passage for references to "amphibians," and find the answer.

4. A

The three physiological zones of the respiratory system are Conducting, transitional, respiratory zones.

5. B

This warranty does not cover a product that you have tried to fix yourself. From paragraph two, "This limited warranty does not cover ... any unauthorized disassembly, repair, or modification. "

6. C

ABC Electric could either replace or repair the fan, provided the other conditions are met. ABC Electric has the option to repair or replace.

7. B

The warranty does not cover a stove damaged in a flood. From the passage, "This limited warranty does not cover any damage to the product from improper installation, accident, abuse, misuse, natural disaster, insufficient or excessive electrical supply, abnormal mechanical or environmental conditions."

A flood is an "abnormal environmental condition," and a natural disaster, so it is not covered.

8. A

A missing part is an example of defective workmanship. This is an error made in the manufacturing process. A defective part is not considered workmanship.

9. B

The first paragraph tells us that myths are a true account of the remote past.

The second paragraph tells us that, "myths generally take place during a primordial age, when the world was still young, before achieving its current form."

Putting these two together, we can infer that humankind used myth to explain how the world was created.

10. A

This passage is about different types of stories. First, the passage explains myths, and then compares other types of stories to myths.

11. B
From the passage, "Unlike myths, folktales can take place at any time and any place, and the natives do not usually consider them true or sacred."

12. A
Based on the partial table of contents, this book is most likely about how to answer multiple choice.

13. B
This passage describes the different categories for traditional stories. The other choices are facts from the passage, not the main idea of the passage. The main idea of a passage will always be the most general statement. For example, choice A, Myths, fables, and folktales are not the same thing, and each describes a specific type of story. This is a true statement from the passage, but not the main idea of the passage, since the passage also talks about how some cultures may classify a story as a myth and others as a folktale.

The statement, from choice B, Traditional stories can be categorized in different ways by different people, is a more general statement that describes the passage.

14. B
Choice B is the best choice, categories that group traditional stories according to certain characteristics.

Choices A and C are false and can be eliminated right away. Choice D is designed to confuse. Choice D may be true, but it is not mentioned in the passage.

15. D
The best answer is D, traditional stories themselves are a part of the larger category of folklore, which may also include costumes, gestures, and music.

All the other choices are false. Traditional stories are part of the larger category of Folklore, which includes other things, not the other way around.

16. A
There is a distinct difference between a myth and a legend, although both are folktales.

17. A
Victoria is about 5 miles from Burnaby.

18. B
The Village Hall is about 5 miles from Victoria.

19. A
Choice A is a re-wording of text from the passage.

20. C
This is taken directly from the passage.

21. C
Although trees are used as a building material, this is not their primary use. Trees are a primary energy source.

22. A
This is taken directly from the passage.

23. D
This question is designed to confuse by presenting different choices for the two chemicals, oxygen and carbon dioxide. One is produced, and one is reduced. Read the passage carefully to see which is reduced and which is produced.

24. B
The correct answer because that fact is stated directly in the passage. The passage explains that Anne taught Helen to hear by allowing her to feel the vibrations in her throat.

25. A
We can infer that Anne is a patient teacher because she did not leave or lose her temper when Helen bit or hit her; she just kept trying to teach Helen. Choice B is incorrect because Anne taught Helen to read and talk. Choice C is incorrect because Anne could hear. She was partially blind, not deaf. Choice D is incorrect because it does not have to do with patience.

26. B
The passage states that it was hard for anyone but Anne to understand Helen when she spoke. Choice A is incorrect because the passage does not mention Helen spoke a foreign language. Choice C is incorrect because there is no mention

of how quiet or loud Helen's voice was. Choice D is incorrect because we know from reading the passage that Helen did learn to speak.

27. D

This question tests the reader's summarization skills. The other choices A, B, and C focus on portions of the second paragraph that are too narrow and do not relate to the specific portion of text in question. The complexity of the sentence may mislead students into selecting one of these answers, but rearranging or restating the sentence will lead the reader to the correct answer. In addition, choice A makes an assumption that may or may not be true about the intentions of the company, choice B focuses on one product rather than the idea of the products, and choice C makes an assumption about women that may or may not be true and is not supported by the text.

28. B

The time limit for radar detectors is 14 days. Since you made the purchase 15 days ago, you do not qualify for the guarantee.

29. B

Since you made the purchase 10 days ago, you are covered by the guarantee. Since it is an advertised price at a different store, ABC Electric will "beat" the price by 10% of the difference, which is,

500 – 400 = 100 – difference in price

100 X 10% = $10 – 10% of the difference

The advertised lower price is $400. ABC will beat this price by 10% so they will refund $100 + 10 = $110.

30. C

The purpose of this passage is to persuade.

31. B

The correct answer can be found in the fourth sentence of the first paragraph.

Option A is incorrect because repenting begins the day

AFTER Mardi Gras. Option C is incorrect because you can celebrate Mardi Gras without being a member of a Krewe.

Option D is incorrect because exploration does not play any role in a modern Mardi Gras celebration.

32. A
The second sentence is the last paragraph states that Krewes are led by the Kings and Queens. Therefore, you must have to be part of a Krewe to be its King or its Queen.

Option B is incorrect because it never states in the passage that only people from France can be Kings and Queen of Mardi Gras. Option C is incorrect because the passage says nothing about having to speak French. Option D is incorrect because the passage does state that the Kings and Queens throw doubloons, which is fake money.

33. C
The first sentences of BOTH the 2nd and 3rd paragraphs mention that French explorers started this tradition in New Orleans.

34. B
Humans have an closed circulatory system.

35. C
Besides blood, the heart and the blood vessels form the cardiovascular system.

Section IV – Basic Science

1. B
The only statement that is NOT true is, Phenotypes are inherited information.

2. D
All of the above are true. Electrons play an essential role in electricity, magnetism, and thermal conductivity.

3. D
An idea concerning a phenomena and possible explanations for that phenomena is an hypothesis.

4. D
All of the above

     a. Structures in a cell nucleus that carry genetic material.
     b. Consist of thousands of DNA strands.
     c. Total 46 in a normal human cell.

5. B
One of the best known disorders that attack the immune system is HIV (the virus that causes AIDS).

6. D
The circulatory system disease that is one of the most frequent causes of death in North America is heart disease.

7. C
The plasma membrane or cell membrane protects the cell from outside forces. It consists of the lipid bilayer with embedded proteins

8. A
The Strong Nuclear Force is an attractive force that binds protons and neutrons and maintains the structure of the nucleus, and the Weak Nuclear Force is responsible for the radioactive beta decay and other subatomic reactions.

Note: The Weak Nuclear Force is so named because it is only effective for short distances. Nevertheless, it is through the Weak Nuclear Force that the sun provides us with energy by allowing one element to change into another element.-

9. D
Qualitative research deals with the quality, type or components of a group, substance, or mixture.

10. A
Adaptation is a trait that has evolved by natural selection.

11. A
A pH indicator measures hydrogen ions in a solution and show pH on a color scale.

12. B
The sun is the earth's primary source of energy.

13. B
The goal of quantitative research is to determine the relationship between one thing (an independent variable) and another (a dependent or outcome variable) in a population.

14. C
A base is any substance that can accept a hydrogen ion and can react with fats to form soaps.

15. D
The dominant gene controls the expression of a trait.

16. B
Plants and animals are kingdoms. There are six recognized kingdoms: Animalia, Plantae, Protista, Fungi, Bacteria, and Archaea.

17. C
Organisms grouped into the Protista Kingdom include all unicellular organisms lacking a definite cellular arrangement such as bacteria and algae.

18. C
Indigestion is a common digestive affliction that most people suffer at one time or other.

19. D
Life functions are the biochemical and biophysical activities that all living systems must be able to carry out to maintain life.

20. C
Angina is frequently mistaken for a heart attack. Angina pectoris, commonly known as angina, is severe chest pain due to ischemia (a lack of blood, thus a lack of oxygen supply) of the heart muscle, generally due to obstruction or spasm of the coronary arteries (the heart's blood vessels). [15]

21. A
A biological class is a collection of similar or like living enti-
ties. Class has the same meaning in biology as rank. Common classes or ranks include species, order, and phylum.

22. A
Fats stay in the stomach the longest.

23. D
The periodic table as it is today, contains 118 elements.

24. D
A Punnett square resembles a game of tic-tac-toe, in which
the genotypes of the   parents gametes are entered first, so
that subsequent combinations can be   calculated.

25. D
All of these statements are true.

> a. Prokaryotic cells include such organisms as E. coli
> and Streptococcus.

> b. Prokaryotic cells lack internal membranes and or-
> ganelles.

> c. Prokaryotic cells break down food using cellular res-
> piration and fermentation.

26. B
The process of converting observed phenomena into data is
called Measurement.

27. A
The mass number of an atom is the total number of particles
(protons and neutrons) that make it up.

28. B
Sublimation is the direct phase transition from solid to gas.

29. A
Exhalation is often accomplished by the abdominal muscles.

30. D
In Eukaryotic cells, the cell cycle is the cycle of events involving cell division, including mitosis, cytokinesis, and interphase.

31. D
All of the choices are correct.

> a. The genetic makeup, as distinguished from the physical appearance, of an organism or a group of organisms.
>
> b. The combination of alleles located on homologous chromosomes that determines a specific characteristic or trait.
>
> c. Is the inheritable information carried by all living organisms.

32. D
The blood is the primarily oxygenated through the work of the respiratory system.

33. B
Ribonucleic acid (RNA) is a chain of nucleotides that plays an important role in the creation of new proteins.

34. A
A practical test designed with the intention that its results will be relevant to a particular theory or set of theories is an experiment.

35. C
Covalent or ionic bonds are considered "strong bonds."

36. A
The process by which the immune system adapts over time to be more efficient in recognizing pathogens is known as acquired immunity.

37. D
An organ is a group of tissues that perform a specific function or group of functions.

38. D
Reliability refers to the measure of an experiment's ability to yield the same or compatible results in different clinical experiments or statistical trials.

39. C
Each chemical element has a unique atomic number representing the number of protons in its nucleus.

40. C
The immune system is the system that protects the body from disease and infection.

41. D
The plasma membrane surrounds the cell and functions as an interface between the living interior of the cell and the nonliving exterior. [15]

42. C
An organelle is a specialized subunit of a cell with a specific function.

43. A
A solution with a pH value of less than 7 is acid. A pH value of 7 is neutral.

44. B
A catalyst is never changed in a chemical reaction.

45. A
The prediction that an observed difference is due to chance alone and not due to a systematic cause; this hypothesis is tested by statistical analysis, and accepted or rejected is the **null hypothesis**.

46. C
In science and engineering, the Accuracy of a measurement system is the degree of closeness of measurements of a quantity to its actual (true) value.

47. B
High blood pressure is a more common name for the circulatory system disease known as hypertension. Hypertension (HTN) or high blood pressure is a cardiac chronic medical condition in which the systemic arterial blood pressure is elevated.

48. B
The range of a distribution is the difference between the maximum value and the minimum value.

49. A
Statistical correlation is a statistical technique which determines if two variables are related.

50. A
In statistical analysis, the mean is the mathematical average of a set of numbers.

51. A
An Atom is the basic or fundamental particle of any matter or element.

52. C
When acid and base react, they neutralize each other properties to form salt and water.

53. B
The horizontal rows from right to left of the periodic table are known as periods and elements on a row share the same number of electron shells.

54. D
Oxidation and reduction reactions are each just half of a redox reaction and both occur simultaneously, because the exact electrons lost in oxidation is what is gained in reduction.

55. B
The elements on the periodic table can be classified as metals, metalloids and non-metals. Most of the elements on the table can be classified as metals.

56. D
All acids contain hydrogen. When acids react with most metals, the metals displace the hydrogen and hydrogen is produced.

57. B
Vertical columns on the periodic table are called groups. There are 18 groups on the table. Elements on the same group each have the same number of electrons on their outermost shell.

58. C
Redox is a complete reaction comprising oxidation and reduction reactions that are each only half of the complete reaction. The same exact electrons lost in oxidation are what are gained in reduction.

59. A
A chemical compound is a chemical substance comprising atoms from two or more elements in a specific ration as expressed in the chemical formula i.e., H2O

60. B
Acids turns blue litmus paper to red, base turns red litmus paper to blue.

Conclusion

CONGRATULATIONS! You have made it this far because you have applied yourself diligently to practicing for the exam and no doubt improved your potential score considerably! Getting into a good school is a huge step in a journey that might be challenging at times but will be many times more rewarding and fulfilling. That is why being prepared is so important.

Study then Practice and then Succeed!

Good Luck!

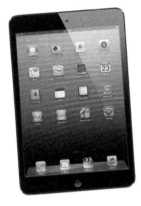

FREE Ebook Version

Go to
http://tinyurl.com/o4v6s3a

Register for Free Updates and More Practice Test Questions

Register your purchase at

www.test-preparation.ca/register.html for fast and convenient access to updates, errata, free test tips and more practice test questions.

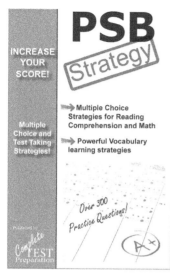

Learn to increase your score using time-tested secrets for answering multiple choice questions!

This practice book has everything you need to know about answering multiple choice questions on a standardized test!

You will learn 12 strategies for answering multiple choice questions and then practice each strategy with over 45 reading comprehension multiple choice questions, with extensive commentary from exam experts!

Maybe you have read this kind of thing before, and maybe feel you don't need it, and you are not sure if you are going to buy this Book.

Remember though, it only a few percentage points divide the PASS from the FAIL students.

Even if our multiple choice strategies increase your score by a few percentage points, isn't that worth it?

https://www.createspace.com/4120266

Enter Code 2KX92YXZ for 25% off!

NOTES

Text where noted below is used under the Creative Commons Attribution-ShareAlike 3.0 License

http://en.wikipedia.org/wiki/Wikipedia:Text_of_Creative_Commons_Attribution-ShareAlike_3.0_Unported_License

[1] Infectious Disease. In *Wikipedia*. Retrieved November 12, 2010 from en.wikipedia.org/wiki/Infectious_disease.

[2] Virus. In *Wikipedia*. Retrieved November 12, 2010 from en.wikipedia.org/wiki/Virus.

[3] Thunderstorm. In *Wikipedia*. Retrieved November 12, 2010 from en.wikipedia.org/wiki/Thunderstorm.

[4] Meteorology. In *Wikipedia*. Retrieved November 12, 2010 from en.wikipedia.org/wiki/Outline_of_meteorology.

[5] U.S. Navy Seal. In *Wikipedia*. Retrieved November 12, 2010 from en.wikipedia.org/wiki/United_States_Navy_SEALs.

[6] Cell Membrane. In *Wikipedia*. Retrieved November 12, 2010 from http://en.wikipedia.org/wiki/Cell_membrane.

[7] Thoracic Diaphram. In Wikipedia. Retrived January 2, 2012 from http://en.wikipedia.org/wiki/Thoracic_diaphragm.

[8] Arrythmia. In Wikipedia. Retrieved January 2, 2012 from http://en.wikipedia.org/wiki/Arrythmia

[10] Emphysema. In Wikipeida. Retreived Jan 2, 2012 from http://en.wikipedia.org/wiki/Emphysema.

[11] Respiratory System. In *Wikipedia*. Retrieved November 12, 2010 from en.wikipedia.org/wiki/Respiratory_system.

[12] Mythology. In *Wikipedia*. Retrieved November 12, 2010 from en.wikipedia.org/wiki/Mythology.

[13] Tree. In *Wikipedia*. Retrieved November 12, 2010 from en.wikipedia.org/wiki/Tree.

[14] Circulatory System. In *Wikipedia*. Retrieved November 12, 2010 from en.wikipedia.org/wiki/Circulatory_system http://www.virtualmedicalcentre.com/anatomy.asp

[15] Angina. In Wikipedia. Retrieved January 20, 2013 from http://en.wikipedia.org/wiki/Angina.